KEEPING CHILDREN *HEALTHY*

The Role of Mothers and Professionals

BERRY MAYALL

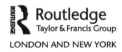

LONDON AND NEW YORK

First published in 1986 by Allen & Unwin (Publishers) Ltd.

This edition first published in 2025
by Routledge
4 Park Square, Milton Park, Abingdon, Oxon OX14 4RN

and by Routledge
605 Third Avenue, New York, NY 10158

Routledge is an imprint of the Taylor & Francis Group, an informa business

© 1986 Berry Mayall

All rights reserved. No part of this book may be reprinted or reproduced or utilised in any form or by any electronic, mechanical, or other means, now known or hereafter invented, including photocopying and recording, or in any information storage or retrieval system, without permission in writing from the publishers.

Trademark notice: Product or corporate names may be trademarks or registered trademarks, and are used only for identification and explanation without intent to infringe.

British Library Cataloguing in Publication Data
A catalogue record for this book is available from the British Library

ISBN: 978-1-041-06510-4 (Set)
ISBN: 978-1-041-01170-5 (Volume 3) (hbk)
ISBN: 978-1-041-01172-9 (Volume 3) (pbk)
ISBN: 978-1-003-61348-0 (Volume 3) (ebk)

DOI: 10.4324/9781003613480

Publisher's Note
The publisher has gone to great lengths to ensure the quality of this reprint but points out that some imperfections in the original copies may be apparent.

Disclaimer
The publisher has made every effort to trace copyright holders and would welcome correspondence from those they have been unable to trace.

KEEPING CHILDREN *Healthy*

The Role of Mothers and Professionals

BERRY MAYALL
*Thomas Coram Research Unit,
University of London*

London
ALLEN & UNWIN
Boston   Sydney

© Berry Mayall, 1986
This book is copyright under the Berne Convention.
No reproduction without permission. All rights reserved.

Allen & Unwin (Publishers) Ltd,
40 Museum Street, London WC1A 1LU, UK

Allen & Unwin (Publishers) Ltd,
Park Lane, Hemel Hempstead, Herts HP2 4TE, UK

Allen & Unwin, Inc.,
8 Winchester Place, Winchester, Mass 01890, USA

Allen & Unwin (Australia) Ltd,
8 Napier Street, North Sydney, NSW 2060, Australia

First published in 1986

British Library Cataloguing in Publication Data

Mayall, Berry
  Keeping children healthy: the role of mothers and professionals.
1. Children – Care and hygiene
I. Title
613'.0432 RJ101
ISBN 0–04–362061–2
ISBN 0–04–362062–0 Pbk

Library of Congress Cataloging-in-Publication Data

Mayall, Berry.
  Keeping children healthy.
1. Children – Care and hygiene. 2. Mothers – Attitudes. 3. Children – Nutrition. 4. Children's accidents – Prevention. 5. Teeth – Care and hygiene. 6. Mothers – Great Britain – Interviews. I. Title.
RJ101.M39
1986   362.1'9892   86–3430
ISBN 0–04–362061–2
ISBN 0–04–362062–0 (pbk.)

Set in 10 on 11 point Sabon by Computape (Pickering) Ltd,
North Yorkshire
and printed in Great Britain by Billing and Son Ltd,
London and Worcester

CONTENTS

Acknowledgements *page* ix

Introduction xi

SECTION A *Setting the Scene*

1 Health Care Work and Inequalities in Health 3

Child Health Care Work 4
Inequalities in Health 9
Class and Health 16
Conclusion 18
Notes to Chapter 1 19

2 The Study 21

The Focus of the Study 21
How We Carried Out the Study 24
Collecting Information from Parents 26
What Kinds of Data Does the Study Provide? 31
What Kind of Status or 'Truth' Does the
   Information Have? 33
How to Deal with the Information 34
Types of Explanation 34
Note to Chapter 2 36

3 Household Resources for Child Health Care 37

The Study Area and the Housing 38
What Kind of Housing Did the Most and
   Least Socially Advantaged Families Have? 42
Income 45
People as a Resource 48

Resources and Health Care	54
Notes to Chapter 3	56

SECTION B *Preventive Care at Home*

4 Safety Care — 59

Introduction	59
Active Children in Poor Housing – a Recipe for Accidents?	60
Keeping Them Healthy as Well as Safe – an Impossible Task?	63
Strategies for Keeping Children Safe	64
Discussion	72
Note to Chapter 4	74

5 Keeping Children Healthy — 75

Introduction	75
What is Good Health?	76
Keeping Children in Good Health	79
Preventing Bad Health	82
Promotion of Health and Prevention of Illness for Children	85
Preventive Care – for Self and Child	86
Mothers' Health Care Work – Implications for Professionals	88

6 Feeding the Children — 90

Introduction	90
What the Children Ate 'Yesterday'	91
Class Differences in Children's Diet 'Yesterday'	96
Income	97
Food Choice – Health and Custom	98
Catering for Children	100
Meals	101
Social Life	103
What Shops Offer	104

	The Daily Round	105
	Obesity	107
	Discussion	109
	Note to Chapter 6	110
7	Caring for Children's Teeth	111
	Introduction	111
	Achieving Good Dental Status	111
	What Happened 'Yesterday'	114
	Tooth-brushing – Who, When and Why Then?	115
	Constraints on Dental Care 'Yesterday'	119
	Help with Dental Care from Professionals	120
	Discussion	123
	Notes to Chapter 7	126

SECTION C *Coping With Illness at Home*

8	Caring for Ill Children	131
	Introduction	131
	Symptoms and Episodes	131
	Class Differences in Illness	133
	Mothers' Knowledge of Children's Illness	134
	Mothers' Care of Ill Children	139
	Why Mothers Contacted the Doctor?	142
	Constraints in Caring for Ill Children	145
	Discussion	149
	Note to Chapter 8	151

SECTION D *Using Health Services*

	Introduction	154
	Health Services in the Study Area	155
	Note to Section D	159
9	Contacts with Health Professionals	160
	Introduction	160
	GPs and Health Visitors	161

	Access to Professional Help	168
	Visits to and from Professionals	172
	Discussion	181
10	Using Preventive Health Services	186
	Introduction	186
	Usage of Preventive Health Services	187
	Discussion	202

SECTION E *Discussion*

11	The Study Reviewed	209
	Preventive Care at Home	209
	Caring for Ill Children and Using Health Services	214
	Knowledge	217
	Control	220
	Responsibility	223
	Notes to Chapter 11	228
12	Helping Mothers Care for Their Children's Health	229
	Introduction	229
	Improving Resources for Health Care	230
	Professionals' Dilemmas	234
	How Professionals Can Help	236

Appendix		241
	Mother's Class	241
	Tables for Appendix	243
Bibliography		251

Acknowledgements

This study was planned and carried out through all its stages collaboratively by two of us at the Thomas Coram Research Unit, myself and my colleague, Chris Grossmith: discussion to focus and refine the study and to construct an interview schedule; carrying out the interviews; and working on the analysis for the book. In particular Chris took responsibility for the analysis of the complex data on symptoms and illness (reported here in Chapter 8). We both gained immensely from working together. I should like to record here my appreciation of his contribution to the project.

I should also like to acknowledge the very great help and support given to us during the course of the study by colleagues at the TCRU, especially Barbara Tizard, Charlie Owen, Ian Plewis and Olwen Davies. I am very grateful to people who read an early draft of the book and spent time helping me with it: Hilary Graham, Ann Oakley, Angus Nicoll, Nancy Kohner and Chris Grossmith. He and I benefited greatly from the help of health authority staff in our area. We could not have done the study without the time, willingness to talk and sympathetic cooperation of 135 mothers. We are especially grateful to them.

Introduction

This book is written with the aim of presenting mothers' perspectives on the health care of their young children. In particular it aims to help health professionals see child health care through mothers' eyes. It is hoped that this perspective may help professionals in their daily work of providing health services for young children and their parents.

The book is based on a study carried out at the Thomas Coram Research Unit. One hundred and thirty-five mothers of first children aged 18–36 months were interviewed and asked about their approaches to health care, their practices and what constrained or facilitated their health care work.

Mothers' health care work takes place within a framework made up of the physical and social world surrounding them. How mothers' behaviour is shaped by their environment is a major theme in the book. For instance the importance of the physical environment is critical, certainly in mothers' eyes, when it comes to safety care. How you keep children safe and how well you can do it depends on characteristics of your housing and your neighbourhood. Also critically important is the quality of the social world of the mother, the child and the family. Women turn to each other for discussion of their children's health and development. What children eat is determined by customs within families, including those handed down from women's own families of origin; it is shaped or, some would say, constrained by the child's social contacts with friends and relatives and at playgroups and minders.

The study showed that the resources – physical and social – that mothers have for health care provide a framework for what they think and do and affect their thoughts and practices. The study was concerned to investigate what these relationships and effects were, for some specific child care topics. So as well as asking mothers about their approaches in general to the health care of their young children, we focused on specific topics: safety care, nutrition and dental care. These were all kinds of care which are likely to have a bearing on the health of the child, and they were also topics which were of interest and importance to mothers. Indeed it was difficult to deal with the wealth of information they gave us.

So a major part of the study was concerned with preventive care at home, what mothers do on a day-to-day basis to maintain and promote their children's health. A second vitally important kind of care mothers give is in monitoring their children for signs of impending illness, and in caring for and treating them when they are perceived to be ill. Almost all the care of ill people, including the care of ill children, takes place out of the public or health professional view, and we aimed to improve understanding of how mothers go about it, what kinds of knowledge they have, and when and why they turn to others for help.

The mothers' accounts of how they keep their children healthy and care for them in illness provide a picture of complex, demanding and absorbing work. Overall, the study suggested that mothers took a highly responsible approach to health care, they had high standards for health in children, and for health care; they dealt with many crises; and their health care work involved constant assessment and choice between priorities. What was also very marked, was that socially disadvantaged mothers had to contend with many more constraints than more fortunate mothers, in caring for their children as they wished.

Setting out to write a book based on an empirical study entails making certain choices about the kind of book it is to be and for whom it is to be written. One approach would be to present the data simply in the form of a research report, setting the study in its social and research context and drawing out some policy implications in a final chapter. Commonly in such books the main interests for the reader are the findings and their relationship to other research findings; the book aims to advance both knowledge and theory within a field. In the case of this study there is no comparable research. The topic of mothers' health care of young children across a socially mixed population has not been studied as a whole – though, as noted throughout this book, there are studies of individual topics, such as nutrition, or use of preventive services. In this book therefore, I chose to emphasize description of mothers' health care work in order to provide a baseline account. It also seemed appropriate to explore and interpret the data. At some points the reader may think comments made are unfounded or inappropriate but it seemed important to point to ideas suggested by the study.

The structure of this book follows the main preoccupations of the study. It starts with an introductory section. This gives an overview of the main issues addressed in the book (Chapter 1). Chapter 2 describes the study – its aims and methods – in some detail. Chapter 3 considers the resources mothers have for their child health work which include characteristics of the housing and the neighbourhood, household income, people available to help with child care, and a potentially important resource – the mothers' educational level.

In Section B, mothers' preventive health care work is considered. First (in Chapter 4), we describe how they keep their children safe. Their perspectives on safety care interconnect with their views on the safety of the housing in the neighbourhood. In Chapter 5 mothers' views on the maintenance of good health and the prevention of poor health are considered and this provides a framework for their more specific approaches to nutrition and dental care (Chapters 6 and 7).

Section C, Chapter 8, describes mothers' work in monitoring their children's symptoms and caring for them when they are ill. Considered together, the five chapters (4–8 inclusive) give an account of health care at home, and they thus provide a natural context for considering use of services.

Section D starts by summarizing some general points about characteristics of health care at home and approaches to health care. These provide a basis for describing and discussing mothers' accounts of their encounters with doctors and health visitors, in Chapters 9 and 10. Mothers' recent use of both curative and preventive health services is described.

In the last section of the book, the study is reviewed and discussed. Suggestions are made at a general level for improving service delivery, bearing in mind always the daily reality of the working lives of parents and professionals.

The book is written mainly for professionals, especially those who help parents with young children: doctors, health visitors and social workers. It is hoped too that it provides a picture of mothers' health care that will interest parents! I have tried to provide a fairly interesting and readable study. I have purposefully not loaded the prose with references, but there is a complete reference list at the end. I have also kept tables in the text to a minimum – a few extra ones have been given in an appendix.

SECTION A

Setting the Scene

1
Health Care Work and Inequalities in Health

This book is about how mothers care for their young children's health. It is about the day-to-day actions they carry out to maintain their children in a healthy state, and about how they look after their children in illness. This is a hidden and neglected topic. Most of mothers' health work for their children takes place at home, out of the public gaze, and much of it is the humdrum stuff of everyday life – feeding them, keeping them away from danger, taking them out for fresh air and exercise. When children are ill, most of the care and treatment is given by mothers at home and only the tip of the illness iceberg is seen by outsiders.

Little attention has been given to mothers' health care work. That could be because it is taken for granted and provides an unconsidered background to the more visible and dramatic work of health professionals in surgeries, clinics and hospitals. In addition, of course, the health care of young children is women's work, and like child care work generally has low status and salience. But mothers' care of their children is important. It is the 24-hour-a-day care they give that largely determines the health, development and welfare of their children. And it is they who decide when, why and for what purposes to seek help from outside the home.

The book draws on a recent study of how 135 London mothers cared for their young children's health. Each of the mothers had a first child aged 18–36 months and the study was concerned to describe how they went about health care – what they thought was important, what they did and what shaped and constrained their actions. It aimed first and foremost to give a broad picture of mothers' health care work, for there has been little systematic study of this: what health care work was like, what mothers had in common in their approaches and practices. The study was also concerned with the issue of inequalities in children's health according to occupational class. It investigated whether there were differences relating to class in mothers' approach to health care, their practices and the constraints and opportunities that affected their practices. Where this was so, it considered whether such differences provided pointers to class differences in children's health and to care and treatment by health professionals.

My colleague Chris Grossmith and myself, both brought practical experience of parenting to the study, but the experience of listening to mothers describing and considering how they cared for their under-threes made us think in different ways than before about this work. Child health care work has some specific characteristics. To set the scene for the book, here are some notes on these.

Child Health Care Work

Health care is women's work. Women care for the health of household members: men, women and children. This remains true in two-parent households, as well as in one-parent households – which are mostly headed by women. It also remains true whether or not women work for money outside or inside the home. The work of health care involves managing household resources to provide food, warmth and clothing; as well as acting directly to promote health, prevent illness and care for ill people (c.f. Graham, 1984).

The daily lives of women who care for young children consist largely of actions that affect health, whether purposefully or not. A trip to the park gives the child exercise, a visit to friends gives the children a chance to play together. Mothers provide food several times a day; dress children according to the weather; watch for signs of illness; pull children away from danger; remember clinic appointments; discuss health and illness with friends and relatives. Some of these actions are taken specifically to promote health. Many are multipurpose, for instance, social life for yourself can at the same time promote the child's social development.

Caring for young children involves constant vigilance and continuous exercise of responsibility. How easy that task is depends on the resources available – other caregivers, characteristics of the physical environment, wealth. With a young child, a mother has to direct the child's actions and provide an environment that will encourage health and prevent ill health, for left to itself the child will come to harm dozens of times a day. Monitoring the child's actions and environment is literally a 24-hour job. Some mothers share these responsibilities with others: fathers and grandmothers take over the task; children may go to playgroup or nursery for a few hours each week. The availability of relatives and friends to share the care probably does not vary by class, but use of pre-school provision certainly does – nationally, and in our sample. More children from socially advantaged households attend pre-school, and from a younger age, than less fortunate children. The environmental resources that facilitate a healthy life for children also vary by class. The well-to-do household in a house and garden can relatively easily provide children with space, fresh air and safety at home; the mother in a cramped dangerous flat has to work very hard and vigilantly to keep the child safe at home, and has to take her out for exercise and fresh air. And the maintenance work of health care is easier if you are well off: going shopping is easier if you have the use of a car; cleaning the home is easier if it is spacious and you have good equipment.

So women caring for young children take many actions that affect the child's health. Some actions are taken specifically to promote health – shielding from danger, nursing a sick child. Others keep the whole household afloat and healthy, such as providing the food or cleaning. There are social activities – maintaining and increasing contacts with friends and relatives. These provide the child with friends too, and help her develop good relationships with relatives. In many circumstances mothers have to choose between competing interests and priorities. A mother may have to take a sick or sleepy child to the shops because she needs food for everyone, though she would prefer to keep the child at home. She may decide to put an unwell child to bed rather than insist on tooth-brushing. She provides food the child will eat, because it will provide nourishment even though it may contain sugar which she thinks is bad for the child's teeth. The child may have to forego her usual two hours at playgroup if the mother has to be at the doctor's with the baby. The child's interests may give way to other people's or theirs to hers depending on what matters most at the time.

A variety of factors enter the decision-making process. Some kinds of health care always take priority. Some circumstances are potentially life-threatening – they always have an urgency and power to divert mothers' attention from any other choices. Mothers will always rush to remove a child from scalding hot water, whatever else is happening. When a child develops a high fever, mothers sit up at night, call taxis, ring sleeping doctors – they take extreme measures and shut out other considerations. Another important factor is what mothers know. Some mothers said they *never* took a child out in winter without head-gear, because they *knew* that would lead to illness. Many routinely provided a main meal of meat and two vegetables because they *knew* that would give children all they needed for health. A third important factor is household patterns. Maintaining family traditions is important, and patterns of behaviour and routines give a framework to the day. The commonest explanation why children's teeth were brushed before, or after, meals, was that 'that's when we do it'. Tooth-brushing was seen as a health care action within the context of household routines.

Of particular interest in this study was mothers' health care when they thought children were in less than perfect health. For a start, these mothers of young children felt they had a direct and immediate insight on when and whether the child was sickening for an illness. They knew what the signs were preceding a child's illness – though these signs might vary between children. Typically they described a child as showing several characteristics that together pointed to illness coming on. Children might look pale, or flushed or heavy round the eyes, or their eyes might look bleary or dulled; they might flop down, refuse to eat, or pick at food, become more attention-seeking or refuse comfort or become whiny or irritable. For the mother, drawing on life-long experience of her child, a particular group of such symptoms had in the past heralded the onset of illness.

An important feature of mothers' interpretation of symptoms is their belief in the *naivety* of the young child's behaviour. These bodily and psychological symptoms are seen as the involuntary reaction of the child to the experience of feeling unwell. As an adult, one may feel that a collection of changes or symptoms in oneself could mean various things: the onset of illness, reaction to stress, unwillingness to face the day's events; and for oneself there remains the question whether to become ill, to adopt the sick role, to succumb, or whether to soldier on, to work one's way through it. Judging from mothers' accounts, they believe there is no such decision-making by small children. The disease comes upon them, and they fall before it, unable to choose not to. This belief among mothers in the direct relationship between the attack of a disease and the child's behaviour helps to explain the spirit in which mothers often seek help. It is often noted that mothers with sick children expect to be given expert help, fast. This may be, not just because children in distress make a fuss one cannot bear to watch, and not just because as a society we think children matter and should go to the front of the queue, but because we believe that the child definitely has something wrong. For ourselves, we may be more dubious, or tentative about seeking help because we are not sure we have anything wrong.

There are other points wrapped up in that paragraph. One is to do with responsibility. Once as a mother you recognize that a child is ill or sickening for illness, you feel you must do something about it: worry, discuss, change management, seek help. You must do something, because the child's welfare, and ultimately her life, is in your hands. For yourself, of course, you may decide to neglect your welfare. It may seem relatively unimportant compared to other priorities like work, social commitments or the child's welfare, or you may be doubtful, as before, of what your symptoms means, or you may know from long experience that neglect will not seriously harm your welfare. But the child is a separate person; you cannot always assess the seriousness of her condition though you know she has one, and you have ultimate responsibility for her life. So you act. Some observers, and probably some mothers, would argue that another factor leading to action is the need or wish to prove to yourself that you have taken responsibility, and further, to be seen by others as responsible (e.g. Locker, 1980).

A second point relating to mothers' perception that the child's behaviour is naive, and to their sense of responsibility, is that they seem to expect health professionals to recognize and respect their perceptions and concerns. The mother reasons first that she knows when the child is ill, secondly that she is responsible for the child, thirdly that her actions are responsible, and fourthly that professionals agree with these points. These assumptions may partly explain why mothers felt it appropriate to summon the doctor from her bed at night, and thought their perception of need for a home visit should be enough to convince the doctor. They explain why mothers were shocked when doctors and nurses questioned their behaviour in taking a child to hospital, or did not respond to their requests to discuss a condition. It seems mothers thought they and health professionals shared an assumption: that parents do their best for their children and so professionals should respond without question to requests for help. But clearly consensus on this point is incomplete. In practice, it seems, the question whether it is for health professionals or for parents to decide when and why parents should receive health service resources (that is, who should ration them) is often decided, or compromised on, by both sides, on the merits of the case.

And, thirdly, accounts of consultations suggest that many health professionals share mothers' feeling of responsibility for children and personal concern for their welfare. This helps to explain why they did respond to requests at 2 a.m., why they urged mothers to bring the child back for a check up after an episode of illness and why they sometimes overrode mothers' wishes. Why professionals feel responsible for children was not a topic considered in the study, though it is good to be able to note that they do! But the issue of the balance of responsibility between parents and professionals for young children's health is a recurring theme.

So child health care work has many specific characteristics. It is largely women's work. Most of the daily activities of women in charge of young children affect children's health, development and welfare, whether intentionally or not. The work involves vigilance and responsibility, but given these it is facilitated by the availability of resources: people to share the care, a good physical environment, sufficient wealth to afford amenities like phones and cars. Mothers have to choose between priorities in health care, and their intimate knowledge of their children helps them to do this. Their knowledge allows them to interpret symptoms and to choose courses of action. Mothers interpret their young children's illness behaviour as naive and feel responsible for their children's welfare; these perspectives lead them to expect a quick, respectful response from health professionals – who in turn often display a sense of responsibility for the children brought to them.

Inequalities in Health

It has been suggested that child health care has some specific characteristics and data from the study will show that mothers had a great deal in common in their approaches to the work. But children's chances of good health in Britain vary according to the circumstances – the socio-economic environment – in which they are born and brought up. The evidence for this continuing situation has been exhaustively assembled and discussed in several recent documents: notably the Court Report (1976), the Black Report (1980),[1] and in Mildred Blaxter's (1981) review. Rather than summarize these reports here, some topics bearing particularly on this study will be noted and discussed.

Perhaps the first point to note is that most of the evidence concentrates on socio-economic advantage and disadvantage as measured by occupational class, though some analyses are available by gender and by gender with class. But evidence is lacking on the compound disadvantages suffered by some ethnic minority people. Disproportionate numbers of them – especially people of Afro-Caribbean or Indian sub-continent background are in low status work, or unemployed; and it is known that in some respects health chances among some groups are poor. For instance, compared to other groups, infant mortality rates are higher where the mothers were themselves born in the Indian sub-continent, West Indies and New Commonwealth Africa (OPCS, 1985); and more mothers from the sub-continent and Africa than others have low birthweight children (OPCS, 1984). It is not known whether and how the two factors – occupational class and ethnicity – interact to produce health status differences. There is widespread feeling among ethnic minorities that institutional racism in the National Health Service (NHS) leads to poor access to services for black people (e.g. Brent CHC, 1981). It is certain that some ethnic minority people suffer from poverty, poor living conditions and from difficulties in getting good services. These factors account for poor health chances for infants and probably for people throughout life, though exactly how is not known. The evidence for inequalities by class conceals inequalities by class *and* ethnicity; and what follows must be understood with that in mind.

The clearest and most final indication of health chances is given in mortality statistics. These give us the tip of the iceberg of ill health. The mortality statistics show that at all stages in life the chances of death increase along the class continuum from class I to class V. And while the death rate for any age group has decreased over the last 60 years, the ratios have remained the same. So, for instance, it could be said for the 1950s that:

> It was as safe in the 1930s to have a baby at home without antenatal care and without specialists to call upon, provided one came from social class I, as it was to have a baby from a social class V background 20 years later.
> (Royal College of General Practitioners, 1982, para. 1.10).

And later on, to put these stark contrasts in numerical terms, if the mortality rates of class I people applied to those in classes IV and V, then in 1970–72 the lives of 74,000 people, including nearly 10,000 children under the age of 15, would have been saved (Townsend and Davidson, 1982, p. 15).

The statistics for young children show that death rates have continued to vary across the years, according to the father's occupational class. Thus, for 1970–72, at birth and in the first month of life, babies whose fathers were in unskilled occupations were twice as likely to die as those with fathers in professional occupations. And in the next eleven months of life the ratios increased: boys were four times as likely and girls five times as likely to die (Black Report, 1980, ch. 2). For children aged 1 to 14 years the death rates also varied by class, though less widely. Boys in class V were twice as likely to die, and girls 1.5 times as likely, as their counterparts in class I.

By the early 1980s – ten years on – death rates in the first year of life had fallen from over 17 to less than 11 per thousand live births. But while there was some variation by class in the rate and direction of changes, overall there was little change in the ratio of deaths in class V compared to class I (OPCS, 1984b).

The main causes of death in the first year of life are congenital malformations, cancers, infections, respiratory conditions, including bronchitis and accidents. And it is the conditions which can be explained most clearly in socio-economic terms which show the steepest class gradients: respiratory conditions and accidents. Respiratory conditions have been linked to family histories of such conditions (so they perpetuate themselves among some groups of people), to number of siblings and to parental smoking and local air pollution. All of these are commoner in socially disadvantaged homes – homes affected by poverty and poor housing. Similarly, accident rates have been linked to local environmental hazards – in housing and the neighbourhood, as well as to children's and adults' behaviour – and these in turn can be explained in terms of people's adaptation to the environment. For older children (aged 1 to 14 years) almost all the class difference in death rates is accounted for by accidents, respiratory conditions, and, to a much lesser extent, by congenital abnormality.

What seems clear from these harsh statistics is that class differences in mortality depend crucially on the child's environment. This includes such factors as housing, pollution levels and danger levels in the neighbourhood, the health of other household members, and the care given by parents. The mortality statistics not only provide an indication of life chances, but point to types of ill health prevalent among children, and to extra ill health among socially disadvantaged children.

The incidence of ill health among children in different class groups has been more difficult to establish from the available sources of information. Much of the data consist of numbers of children receiving medical attention, or of survey data from mothers, and both of these could be subject to class-related behaviours or perceptions. While the evidence of class difference is less clear-cut, however, the general tendency of findings from many studies is to show that amounts and severity of ill health are greater among socially disadvantaged children (Blaxter, 1981, ch. 6). The large-scale surveys such as the Newcastle Study, the National Survey of Health and Development and the National Child Development Study (NCDS) have all found more respiratory conditions, especially serious ones, among these children than their more fortunate contemporaries.[2] And the NCDS, which examined children at age seven, found evidence of class differences in several aspects of health and development. For instance, more children in socially disadvantaged homes than of others had histories of middle ear infections and more had squints and unhealthy teeth (Davie, Butler and Goldstein, 1972). On the other hand, the evidence from the annual survey of reported illness in the General Household Survey does not show a consistent trend. However, it does seem that the reported number of visits to doctors does not match the general pattern of extra ill health among class IV and V children. And it has consistently been shown over many years that these children are taken less often to preventive health services, so their health and progress are less fully overseen by medical staff (Cartwright and O'Brien, 1976; Graham and McKee, 1980). However, it is possible that things are changing. Moss, Bolland and Foxman (1982) found no class differences in clinic attendance over the first year (though they had few households from the 'lower' working classes). The large-scale Child Health and Education in the Seventies (CHES) study carried out on children born in 1970 showed that use of clinic services by age five, did not differ by class – though immunization rates did.[3] It seems therefore that the incidence of ill health – particularly serious ill health – increases along the class continuum and that usage of curative services is lower than might be expected. Usage of preventive services has traditionally been lower, but this may be changing. It has also been argued, and demonstrated, that services for the poor are likely to be poor services (Tudor Hart, 1971; Skrimshire, 1978).

Explanations for class differences in health – the debate

But why do these sharp class differences in health persist and what kinds of explanation account for them? For a start, if there is a health service freely available to all, why is it that all do not have an equal chance of health? It seems that the provision of the NHS has not in itself served to ensure that people have good health. This could be in part because, as suggested above, there is disparity in the services offered to people in 'poor' areas and those offered in the well-to-do areas. Apart from that factor, however, there are two main types of explanation proposed.

At one extreme on a long continuum stand the structuralists. According to their account, general ill health can be seen as an effect of poverty. People's low income, poor housing and poor working conditions directly cause ill health. Less directly, the circumstances in which poor people typically live their lives are thought to affect their health adversely. Thus people in insecure, poorly paid work cannot easily take time off to rest or seek help when they are ill; people living in a stressful environment may smoke to get through the day; mothers with many children and the burdens of paid work, poor housing and inadequate help may neglect both their own and their children's health; mothers living under those circumstances may find it more difficult to breast-feed their babies (assuming that is a good thing) than those with leisure and help around the house. Finally, on this theme, it is argued that social distance between health professionals and 'lower' working class people, and the latter's low levels of education, inhibit their access to knowledge of good health behaviour. In other words, it is suggested that on at least some important topics, top people know what behaviours lead to good health and furthermore are structurally able to change their life-style and adopt them. Supporting evidence for this is the early adoption by middle class mothers of breast-feeding and non-smoking, once the arguments were presented to them.

At the other end of the continuum stand those who, while admitting the relevance of some of this, take essentially a behavioural or individualist stance. They argue that most individuals in whatever social circumstances do have the ability to behave well — that is, in ways that professionals think appropriate for ensuring good health. People who cannot or will not behave like the majority may be described as inadequate in terms of their personality. Thus Tonge, James and Hillam (1975) studied 'problem families' and having noted their poverty, poor housing and the recurrent crises which beset them (such as unemployment and illness) argued that they were distinguished by pathological deviations from normal perceptions and behaviour. Another kind of interpretation can be, simply, in terms of deprivation. Such people lack both knowledge and the acquired life-styles that would facilitate good behaviour and hence health, but they can be taught to know and do better, within their existing social circumstances.

It will be noted that when we talk about 'good' behaviour we run up against assumptions about the sort of society we live in. It can be argued that it is one with largely shared values; individuals and groups do more or less well in adhering to them. Or it can be argued that it is a society made of many sub-cultures, each with its own worth and none widely accepted as the norm. When considering leisure pursuits, or attitudes to paid work, or values in child rearing, you can readily produce an argument for either vision of how it is we think about our society. But when it comes to health, there seems little doubt that there are some dominant values, beliefs and pieces of knowledge; they tend to be held by health professionals, who may argue fine points among themselves, but who present an influential vision of how people should behave. Those who behave differently may be stigmatized, and encouraged to conform. Furthermore, types of health behaviour gain approval and disapproval according to their acceptability by this dominant group. For example, most people risk their own and others' health in various ways, but it is the risky actions associated with working class people that are highlighted. Thus campaigns against smoking and for breast-feeding and wearing seat belts rank high on the health education agenda, whereas campaigns against people who drive fast cars or send young children to residential institutions (prep schools!) do not.

Presenting structuralist and behaviouralist stances thus briefly and schematically may help one think about explanations for class inequalities in health. But to do so diverts attention from other important points. One is the argument that health status itself is a major determinant of class status; those in poor health tend to end up in low status jobs; so there is a social drift downwards of those in poor health and these tendencies help explain the extra prevalence of poor health in the 'lower' classes. A further important point is that various mixes of approaches probably serve best to explain class inequalities, and which mix fits best depends on what topic is being considered. Thus many commentators agree that while adult and child behaviour is relevant to accident rates in children, the physical environment probably matters most. But people are probably less well agreed on what factors, material or behavioural, are likely to lead to heart attacks. Probably social drift does partly 'explain' some characteristics of some people who live in doss houses, but various interactions of material and behavioural factors are no doubt relevant too (see Thomson, 1984).

In part, of course, people's perspectives on explanations for class differences in ill health reflect the work they do. Those whose work is with individuals – helping them care for their health (like nurses, doctors and health visitors) or helping them cope in disadvantaged environments (like case workers in social work) are likely to feel that individual people do have the capacity to make life better for themselves and their dependants, within the unchanging circumstances of their environment. They observe in their daily working lives that some individuals do rise above their circumstances, some are more eager than others to listen, learn and change. So workers in the 'caring' professions may favour explanations for inequalities in health that are

Health Care Work and Inequalities in Health 15

behavioural rather than structuralist. Thus studies of 'problem families' in the 1960s and 1970s arose from the practical aim of the social work profession to help people in the here and now. Sociological theory was invoked to justify intervention at the level of people's functioning, even where social and material circumstances remained the same. They could be helped to give their children better care, to manage their incomes, to hold down jobs and to improve personal relationships. Similarly, the Royal College of General Practitioners (RCGP), having surveyed the evidence for class inequalities in children's health, has proposed a programme of health education by GPs, directed at parents (RCGP, 1982, 1984).

> Even more important than physical environment is the emotional environment. People are more important than places. The health and happiness of the child is dominated by the attitudes, values and relationships of the family.
>
> (RCGP, 1984, para. 2.11).

The professional aim of changing individuals rather than circumstances is justified by an appeal to theory: people matter more than places; parents can do well for their children even in poverty and poor housing. So while these documents recognize material constraints on parents' chances of seeing their children growing up healthy, they nevertheless argue that parents should assume more responsibility than many do for their children's health. And they see changes in parental behaviour as the key to children's health chances.

It is not part of the argument of this book that people are powerless to change their behaviour because of their environmental constraints. Rather the book suggests that the implication that people's willingness to do well for their children varies by class, is a misconstruction or misinterpretation of the available evidence. The argument of the book is that mothers' health care of their children is not very different according to class. Mothers are much more similar across the class groups than they are different. Their approaches to health related child care, and the purposes of what they do for their children – keeping them healthy in the context of other responsibilities and of constraints – are much the same. To the extent that their practices vary by class these variations can be explained in terms of knowledge and practical material constraints and opportunities. Study findings do not suggest that any groups of mothers are unwilling to do well for their children. Indeed it would be strange if mothers did differ by class in their approaches to health related child care. What they have in common as mothers is stronger than what differentiates them.

It should also be said here that the findings of the study described in this book tend to support the argument advanced in the Black Report (Townsend and Davidson, 1982, ch. 6): it is in some version of the structural explanation that the best explanations for class differences in health and health care lie, at least as far as children are concerned. This is not to say that behavioural or cultural explanations do not have relevance and force in particular circumstances, as later chapters will show.

Furthermore, it is a major thesis of this book that at a policy level it is inappropriate to accept the theory of behavioural change without addressing the fundamental structural inequalities which shape the environment within which people rear their children. While behaviour may be affected in some cases and in some areas of child health care, such behavioural changes are unlikely to make a major difference to the health chances of children living in poverty-stricken households where people have poor housing, poor neighbourhoods and poor prospects.

Class and Health

So far, the word 'class' has been used without comment on its meaning, and on its force as a discriminator between groups of people. For while class is a good discriminator of differences in health status and health chances it does not itself provide an explanation of these differences. Indeed the explanation for differences revealed in analyses by class has to be sought in the many factors that go to make up what is pointed to when we classify people according to their occupation – that is, such factors as income, education, housing, neighbourhood, life-style. If we are thinking of how children do or do not achieve good health, then it is by considering a range of such factors that we are likely to find convincing explanations for class differences. Furthermore, one kind of factor may be particularly important in certain areas of health care; thus housing may affect safety care and the chances of accident; but the child's own history of respiratory illness may be more relevant in explaining characteristics of the care of that child when she is ill.

So if we are concerned with health care given by mothers, how helpful is it to consider households divided into groups according to occupation? And whose occupation? The grading of people according to occupation was first systematized by the Registrar General in 1911. The classification of occupational categories was constructed such that it pointed to group differences in mortality. The system distinguishes between groups of people according to the degree of skill and social position implied in their occupation, which in practice broadly covers their income, education, housing and life-style (Leete and Fox, 1977). It is a grading conceived for men's work, rather than for women's. When men are graded according to the Registrar General's classification, the ranking does commonly serve to distinguish broadly between groups of households according to factors indicating levels of advantage. Generally men in high status jobs have high incomes, high levels of education, good housing in pleasant neighbourhoods, compared to those further down the social ladder. So the Registrar General's is a useful classification in that it is a recognizable clue to levels of affluence, and 'social standing'. It points to the health hazards associated with occupational class. It is also useful because, since it is widely used, it allows for the findings of one study to be compared with those of another.

A major disadvantage of the grading is that it gives inadequate recognition to characteristics of women's work and their contribution to household affluence and life-styles. If classified according to the Registrar General women tend to fall into two large groups: those in class II in professional and managerial work such as teaching, social work and nursing; and those in class III in non-manual work such as office work, or in manual work such as skilled trades and factory work. The rating does not recognize different levels of skill and seniority within women's work, nor the range of income, and nor does the rating for women put them into groups comparable in affluence or status with those for men.

There are at least two other respects in which the Registrar General's classification has to be treated with caution. First, it is not always a very good discriminator for young people, whose type of work may vary widely over a short space of time, and whose level of affluence may not 'fit' with the description of the majority in their class group. You can be very poorly off as a young lawyer (class I) or teacher (class II) compared to most people in those classes. Secondly, the grading does not cope with the unemployed, who are excluded from the rating, and who are usually reclassified according to their previous job, or their main job. The levels of affluence in many households are crucially affected by benefits of various kinds – housing subsidies, unemployment benefit and the like, and these effects are concealed when an unemployed carpenter or teacher is assigned to their previous occupation.

In our study, we tried to take account of the advantages and disadvantages of using the Registrar General's classification. We used it to group the households, according to the father's job, because we wanted comparability with other studies and large scale figures. But we also collected data on mothers' work, on income, on housing and the neighbourhood environment, and on fathers' and mothers' educational level, including, for mothers, their training and qualifications for work. So we were able to use these variables, singly or grouped, to set against findings.[4]

A second reason for settling on this classification was that for this sample income, housing, the neighbourhood environment and mother's education were closely correlated with the father's class according to the classification. So his class provided a good indicator of levels of advantage in these respects. However, while those households with fathers in high status jobs were almost all advantaged in respect of housing and mother's education, for those in classes III, IV and V the correlations were not quite so close. In other words there was more variation in housing conditions and in mother's education. So it was sometimes possible for households in these classes (though not for those in classes I and II) to show that income or mother's education was independently related to certain aspects of child health care. In addition, because we wanted to take account of mothers' part in determining health care practices in the household we devised a class we called 'Mother's class' which took account of her educational level (see Chapter 3).

Conclusion

This chapter has introduced some of the major issues considered in this book. Two topics are perhaps salient and give particular cause for thought.

First, the work of keeping children healthy is a demanding, complex and highly responsible job. Those who deal professionally with mothers who do this work need to consider what the implications of its characteristics are for their own work and for their interactions with mothers. What kind of service should professionals offer to mothers? Should it be interventionist or responsive to what mothers want? Is it appropriate for professionals to think in terms of educating mothers, and should they aim to learn from mothers? How is responsibility for children best shared between parents and professionals?

Secondly, it is clear from the research evidence that whatever other factors may be relevant, material disadvantage is implicated as an important factor leading to early death, accident and illness. We are living in a society where material disadvantage, far from decreasing, is on the increase. Unemployment, housing policies and reductions in benefits are obliging millions to live in poverty. It has been estimated that a third of our children are now being brought up in poverty (Piachaud, 1981b). At the same time services are being cut back, so that people find, for instance, there is deterioration in the quality of health service care, and fewer and poorer day-care services for under-fives even compared with the miserly provision of the 1970s. Professionals – health visitors, doctors and social workers – stand between these two forces, the increase in poverty and the contraction of services. How should they respond to the challenge? For instance, health visitors who have traditionally valued and given a universalist service to families with under-fives, are now debating whether concentration on disadvantaged families may be not only a matter of day-to-day exigency but preferable. Some professional people are taking a more political, or welfare rights, approach to their work, and offering practical help rather than education or case work.

These themes will be taken up and discussed throughout the book in relation to study findings. The next chapter goes on to describe the study, its aims and methods.

Notes to Chapter 1

1 The Black Report came out in 1980. It was the report of a committee set up by the then Labour Government, under the Chairmanship of Sir

Douglas Black. Other committee members were Professor Peter Townsend, Professor J. N. Morris, Dr Cyril Smith. It was not made widely available. An abridged version was published in 1982, under the authorship of Townsend and Davidson. It is mainly this version that is referred to in this book.

2 The Newcastle study of 1,000 families took a random sample of children born in 1947 in the city and monitored them through childhood (e.g. Spence *et al.*, 1954).

The NSHD took over 5,000 children born in 1946 and has followed them through to adulthood (e.g. Douglas and Blomfield, 1958).

The National Child Development Study has followed all children born in a week in March 1958 in England, Wales and Scotland through childhood (e.g. Davie, Butler and Goldstein, 1972).

3 The Child Health and Education in the 1970s study (CHES) is a longitudinal study of all children born in the UK in one week in 1970, carried out under the direction of Neville Butler. Data referred to here come from an unpublished report on the children's physical health and use of services, over their first five years entitled: 'From Birth to Five'.

4 Because we thought grouping households by class might not serve to group them according to social advantage we also tried out the Social Index devised for the CHES study which gives a broad measure of advantage based on: father's job, the highest level of education reached by either parent, and housing characteristics (crowding, tenure, type of housing) and a rating of the neighbourhood (Osborn and Morris, 1979). For the purposes of our study we adapted their measure of neighbourhood environment to fit the area under study, because their measure did not discriminate between good and bad environments in our area. However, this revised social index correlated very closely indeed with both father's and mother's class, and was not useful in providing a means of discriminating between households independently of class. So in the event, the Social Index was not useful for this study.

2

The Study

The Focus of the Study

The evidence assembled and discussed by the Black Committee and by Mildred Blaxter shows that there are large differences in children's health chances in Britain today, indeed in their chances of survival, and it is consistently children from socially advantaged backgrounds who have the best chances. In addition the evidence is that ill health in childhood may cast long shadows forward. Unhealthy children may become unhealthy adults. There seems little doubt that explanations for class inequalities in child health are urgently needed. In this chapter the aims and methods of the study are described and discussed. Detail is given to satisfy some readers. Others may wish to skip all or most of the chapter!

When we began to plan a study on child health we decided to focus on children's *access* to health and to health services, through the care their parents give them. We planned to study, not so much how healthy the children were, as how their parents looked after their health. We thought it important to investigate the main setting, or context, in which children's health is maintained or restored. Most children spend most of their early years in the charge of one or two parents at home. In practice the mother is usually the main caregiver. So how healthy the children are depends largely on the care she, or they, give. Looking at it from the parents' point of view, the health services are services parents call on among other sources of help, when they consider they need them. Yet studies taking this parental perspective are few (e.g. Luker, 1975; Buswell, 1983) compared to the vast majority which start from the perspective of the health services or of health service staff, and ask how well parents or consumers or patients fit in with what is provided, or behave as professionals deem appropriate. Thus a study may start with health professionals' concern that some parents do not bring children to be checked over at the child health clinic or to be immunized. From a professional standpoint it may seem obvious that parents should do so. When parents do not use services, they may be castigated as 'defaulters', 'low attenders', even as 'poor parents' and reasons for their 'non-compliance' sought. But the situation may look quite different if the parental perspective is the starting point. Parents may not see it as part of their job to take children to be checked over and immunized, or they may think it is their responsibility to decide what actions to take on behalf of their child. There may in fact be a mismatch between parental and professional perspectives. Studying child health care from a parental perspective may further understanding of how they see their task, and may help professionals to respond appropriately and effectively to these perspectives.

The reader will have noticed that use of the word 'parent' strikes a discordant note in the above. As we all know, it is mothers who care for young children, who use services for children and get the blame if children do not attend for check-ups. But in planning the study we thought fathers might be in charge in some families, and tried not to make assumptions about the principal caregiver's sex.

What we wanted to know about

We aimed to study a series of related questions. The first set of questions was concerned with what parents perceived to be the job of caring for their children's health. What did they see as their health care responsibilities? What did they believe to be important health care practices? What did they actually do to maintain their children's health? What did they perceive as helping or hindering them in this work of health care? We were aiming here to provide a description of parental health care. This is a topic that has not received much research attention. We know of only one study that has addressed directly these questions – Blaxter and Paterson's (1982) useful study of working class mothers in Aberdeen. There have been some studies which have covered the transition to parenthood, and have focused on parental perspectives; these have covered pregnancy and the early months of first-time parenting and the emphasis has been on how well services help parents, and on what child care problems parents meet (e.g. Moss, Bolland and Foxman, 1982; Graham and McKee, 1980). We decided to focus on the care of slightly older children, so that parents would be well into the swing of parenthood, and would have ideas derived from experience about caring for children's health.

The second set of questions was about what parents perceived to be the usefulness of health services in helping them care for their children's health. How well did health services suit the needs and wishes of parents for their children? What sorts of qualities in health professionals did parents like and dislike? Under what circumstances and for what purposes did parents use health services, and which ones did they use for what? Why did they choose not to use some health services, for instance preventive ones? By providing information on these topics we hoped to contribute to explanations of why some groups of children are overseen by the services while others have less contact. Such explanations might help professionals understand parental motivation for use or non-use and help them respond appropriately when planning services and relating to parents.

We also wanted to know whether there were differences between groups of parents: in their approaches to child health care; in their practices; and in what factors affected their practices. Were there differences between groups in their use of health services, in their satisfaction with services and in their opinions of them? The question here was, if there were differences between groups of parents, were these associated with such factors as housing, levels of affluence, quality of social networks. If occupational class strongly and persistently seemed to distinguish groups, was it possible to unpack it into constituent factors such as housing or affluence and was it possible to show that such factors had an explanatory power independently of class?

Finally, we wanted to contribute to the debate: did the weight of the evidence contribute to the debate about structuralist versus behavioural explanations for inequalities in health?

So we aimed to study how parents cared for their children's health at home, their use of health services for their children, and the extent to which class, and factors associated with class served to account for differences in health care. We planned the study so that we could consider these topics.

How We Carried Out the Study

Choosing the households and the area

We chose an area no more than two miles across in any direction with households living in it from the full range of occupational classes. We identified households living in the area by a door-to-door survey and included into our sample only those households which met a set of criteria. Each household had a mother who was white and born in the British Isles; she lived with her husband or boyfriend – and she had a first child aged 18–36 months. We found 165 households who met these limited criteria, out of 15,500 households in the area. Of these 165, 8 per cent were unwilling to take part in the study and 10 per cent moved away before we could interview them. In the end we had 135 interviews – 82 per cent of the possibles. According to the father's present or most recent job (Registrar General) the households fell into two broadly equal groups. Forty-one per cent were in professional or managerial work and another 7 per cent in skilled non-manual work; so 48 per cent were in 'non-manual' work. Fifty-two per cent were in skilled (33 per cent) semi-skilled (14 per cent) or unskilled (5 per cent) work. (The class divisions of the sample are further discussed in Chapter 3).

The restriction of the sample by a set of criteria meant that in some important respects the households were similar to each other. They were all two-parent households and they were all caring for a first child who was past babyhood, but not yet, in most cases, spending much time away from her parents and home. This is a time in the child's life when parents have perhaps less help than for a baby in that there is less intervention by services. So parents would have had the time to develop ideas from experience about child health care, probably took most of the decisions themselves, but were all doing this for the first time.

Having a restricted sample was an important part of the design because it would help us to consider the significance of what we found. If we wanted to compare groups of households we would be to some extent comparing like with like. Interpretation would not be confused by the presence of other variables – such as several older children, or the presence of only one parent in the household.

So in this study we conducted a limited exercise in the interest of answering some specific questions about class differences. We chose to exclude many people who make up class groups, such as those with several children, lone-parent households and ethnic minority households. Class differences in health as shown in the statistics stem at least partly from the fact that semi-skilled and unskilled workers' households (Registrar General classes IV and V) are made up disproportionately of households such as these, which by and large are severely constrained by material and social disadvantage. Our resources limited the size of the sample. Had we included in our sample of 130–40 households all those in an area with a child in a given age-range, we would have been able to describe the wide variety of types of household which go to make up class groups as defined by the Registrar General. And we could have described their health care of their young children. But we could not have made any attempt to account for health care practices in terms of constraining and facilitating factors, because the number and complexity of these would have been too great to make sense of. Furthermore, to give each interviewee an equal chance of talking adequately about the topics concerned, we would have needed a very large research team with people who spoke the many relevant languages. In other words, the research project would have had to be much bigger and more expensive in terms of time and staffing than was feasible.

As noted in Chapter 1, it is clear that people in ethnic minorities suffer poorer health chances, including poor access to services, than other people. The problem for the research worker is to offer a useful contribution to understanding the interplay and importance of various factors, poverty, powerlessness inherent in occupational class position and racism. Similarly women (and to a lesser extent men) heading lone-parent families are very likely indeed to suffer from poverty, to be restricted to low status jobs or no jobs at all and to meet prejudice. Limiting the number and kinds of people included in a study is necessary in the interests of trying to address some questions systematically, but it involves difficult choices. In this case, the study was seen as a first stage study in health care. It is planned to address questions on ethnicity and resources for health care in a second study.

The area for the study was chosen partly because it had a good mix of households by class, and was reasonably accessible to the interviewers, and partly because households living there had much the same set of reasonably good child health services. There seemed little point in studying parents' views of services that most customers and professionals would condemn. We assumed, that is, that some characteristics of services were good. Some areas we considered had child health clinics housed in church halls – they looked to us inconvenient, inhospitable and drab; hospitals were far away – even by bus or train. The area finally chosen was in inner North London. It was the catchment area of two district health authority health centres, purpose-built, with clinics housed there. There were two hospitals within a maximum of a half hour's walk for any parent in the area. The health services are described later, when mothers' usage of them is considered (see Introduction to Section D).

Collecting Information from Parents

We had identified our area and the households we wanted to include in the study. There were important decisions to be made about how best to collect information from parents about their perceptions of child health care. We decided that since the study was about what parents' perceptions on health care and on health services were, it was appropriate to interview them and get them to talk about these topics. Perhaps the other broad option would have been to try to observe parental health care and use of services, but this is a very time-consuming method and might well not have been acceptable to the people concerned. Nor would it have covered all the topics we wanted to cover.

We aimed to interview the parent who provided day-to-day care. When we called at the home to ask parents to take part we asked who did this. Since it was usually the mother who answered the door, we may have got an unduly mother-biased view. But only 2 fathers (out of 135) were caring for their children full-time during the day, and although some fathers and mothers told us that the fathers did more than 'help' in that they took a *share* of the child-care, it was clear from the interviews that traditional patterns prevailed. Though some mothers did paid work (mostly part time) child care was the mothers' main province and responsibility, and paid work with some child care in some cases was the fathers' province. Once we had established who was the main caregiver we asked for an interview and in practice, in most cases, saw the mother alone. Some fathers (29 per cent) were present some of the time: some dropped in casually but others probably chose to be there because the two parents in these households saw themselves as sharing child-care responsibilities fairly evenly, and as both having something to contribute to an interview about parental care of young children. So in these cases while we tried (for the sake of consistency) to get the mother's perceptions and accounts we did not hinder parents from discussing points with each other.

The other main decision was whether to interview once, or more than once. In earlier studies we had found that you get more reliable information if you ask about fairly recent events, and we thought about visiting twice or more to collect two or more sets of recent events. In the end we decided that given the time we had, interviewing more people once would give us better information about patterns of child care across different groups of parents, than interviewing fewer people more than once. It was also important to think about the interview from the mother's viewpoint. Visiting more than once is time-consuming for the researcher, but it may also be inconvenient, difficult and in the end unacceptable, for mothers. It may mean that some drop out of the study, so that you have incomplete sets of information from some mothers. So in the end we settled on doing one longish interview with each mother (in two cases the father, and in a few cases both parents).

We also considered asking mothers to fill in with us a health diary of recent events and perceptions. We tried this out. Mothers enjoyed doing it with us and it produced vivid information, but since in the recent past nothing of central interest to us had happened in some households, we would have to collect diaries on several occasions from each household to be sure of getting a reasonable amount of information that could be compared across groups of mothers. We also considered leaving diaries with mothers to fill in, but rejected this approach because we wanted detailed, elaborated information – and we could not expect mothers to sit down and write lengthy paragraphs about the day's events.

The interview schedule

We devised an interview schedule to cover a range of health care topics. We included enough topics so that we could look across them and see if patterns of health care emerged. But we restricted the number of topics so that we could cover each in some detail. And we focused the interview on the 'focus' child – the first child aged 18–36 months. So all data reported in this book on 'the children' relates to those first children. We asked some mothers to help us by trying out with us early versions of the schedule and in the light of these experiences we drew up a final version. This covered mothers' ideas and practices on promoting their children's health, preventing illness, safety care, feeding the child and dental care. We asked what symptoms led them to think the child was ill, what actions they took to care and treat ill children and whether they sought any help from health professionals or from friends and relatives. We also covered recent contacts with the doctor and health visitor, visits to hospitals and visits to the clinic for preventive care, and, looking further back, whether children had been taken for developmental checks and for immunization. In addition we collected some background information – for instance on parents' work, mother's education, housing and income, contacts with relatives and friends.

So the interview focused on preventive care at home, on the care of ill children at home and on the use of health services. For each of the preventive care topics we adopted the same approach. We asked mothers what they thought important, what were their priorities, what they actually did, and what sorts of factors they thought influenced what they did. The method was to introduce a topic with a broad question, to encourage the mother to start talking about it, and to add in prompt questions to cover points we thought important. Similarly, when asking about the care of ill children and contact with health professionals, we asked the mother to give us an account of what had happened, and had ready a list of prompts in case she didn't cover them.

Doing the interviews

At our initial approach to the mothers, to ask them for an interview, we explained that the interview would take over two hours. Perhaps it is a measure of how compelling the subject is for mothers that very few (8 per cent) preferred not to take part in the study. We arranged with the mother a time when she could give us that much time, during the day or the evening; sometimes the child was present, sometimes not. The interviews varied in length; most took 2 to 2½ hours (32 per cent) or 2½ to 3 hours (44 per cent). A few (8 per cent) took longer when mothers had a lot to say or when various events interrupted the interview. In a few cases (16 per cent) the interview had to be done in a shorter time (under two hours) because something cropped up to prevent the mother from giving more time to it. The interviews were carried out in the first nine months of 1982.

The two of us who planned out the study and wrote the schedule did the interviews. So we knew what broad questions we wanted answers to and from the outset we knew the detail of the schedule well enough to give mothers the freedom to talk about topics as and when they wished. In order to lessen chance bias in who did which interviews we stratified the sample by class and then randomly assigned ourselves half the sample each, within class groups. So each of us did a socially mixed half of the interviews.

Our own background knowledge of health was an important factor in the way we approached mothers. Both of us were parents and had first-hand experience of caring for children's health. Neither of us had any medical training, that is, we had not been through courses such as those for trainee doctors and nurses. Our health knowledge and approaches to health were in that sense 'lay'. We explained these points to mothers. In addition, we were able in honesty to tell them at the outset that we aimed to find out what they thought was important in health care; we were not trying to test them to see if they had 'correct' ideas and practices according to health professionals' perspectives. We were also able to say that we had no connection with any health service, but came from a research unit which traditionally sought to identify and promote parents' perspectives. We explained that we aimed to learn what mothers do for their children's health, so that we could offer this information to health professionals to help them understand parents' perspectives and give parents appropriate and responsive help.

These explanations were important to justify the research to mothers and to establish that we were seriously interested in hearing their perspectives. The explanations also served, at least somewhat, to lessen the inevitable distance between us (interviewers) and them (mothers). For the interview was not between professionals or knowledgeable people on one side and lay or less knowledgeable people on the other. It was between people who in an important sense were on the same side – that of recognizing and promoting the reality and value of mothers' perspectives.

A second kind of difference between research interviewer and interviewed is often to do with class. Reseachers usually have some characteristics that differentiate them from some groups of interviewees, characteristics associated (in *all* our minds?) with class: relatively high levels of education, possibly manner, evidence of relative affluence. Up to a point, we thought the common interests identified above provided a bridge across these differences. And we felt we got on well with most mothers in all class groups; with most we established an easy, seemingly open relationship. However, it is possible that in classes III, IV and V some women's answers and stories were affected by the perceived class gap between them and us. So they may have told us what they thought we wanted to hear; or concealed, more than other mothers, aspects of the 'truth' as they saw it.

Our feeling about the interviews with the 135 mothers was that in all but a handful of cases they were relaxed and felt free to talk openly about their ideas and practices. They were not trying to give standard or 'correct' answers. Once they understood that we really did want to hear about the detail of their beliefs, their practices and what helped or hindered them in caring for their children's health, they were keen to talk. In addition, we had going for us the fact that mothers enjoy talking about the details of child care and we were offering them the (rare) opportunity of talking at length to eager listeners who did not want to interrupt with their own stories.

We wanted as full an account as possible of how mothers cared for their children's health and a complete record of what they said. So we asked to tape-record the interviews. Most mothers thought this was quite acceptable. The interviewer transcribed the tape-recording immediately after the interview. In the half-dozen cases where the mothers disliked the idea we wrote full notes of what they said, during the interviews.

We coded the interviews. The coding took into account what was said at each point of the interview but it also included summary codes that drew together what mothers had said on a topic from any part of the interview. When all the interviews were done we reconsidered the coding in the light of experience.

During the course of the work we took various steps to make reasonably sure that the two of us were doing the interviews, and coding the interview findings, in the same way. We had worked on the schedule together and agreed on what we were trying to find out. We each practised the interviews and discussed procedures and problems. Then we did a series of practice interviews together and discussed methods and difficulties. We held a weekly meeting during the main interviewing period to discuss how we were doing the interviews, any problems that arose and coding problems. Finally, we checked through each other's coding of the findings and discussed and sorted out discrepancies and problems.

What Kinds of Data Does the Study Provide?

All the information obtained was given by the 135 mothers during an interview, except for some background points about characteristics of local health services, which we obtained from district health authority staff.

It is *systematic information*, in the sense that everyone was asked the same questions. It is also systematic in the sense that we had an end in view and collected certain sorts of data towards that end. As noted earlier, we limited the focus of the study in the interests of getting detailed information, and for each health care topic studied we collected information on beliefs, practices and factors that affected these. We were then able to compare these across topics and could attempt to identify patterns across all of what one mother said and patterns common to groups of mothers. Thus we could compare what they said about factors leading to good dental health and about factors leading to good general health. We could see links between mothers' ideas about healthy children and their problem in keeping them safe: they thought a healthy child was active and exploratory, and they therefore wanted to provide an environment that both gave opportunities for active play and was safe – a difficult task in urban housing. The study also allowed us to set mothers' use of services against what we learned of their perspectives on health care at home. We began to see why mothers rushed off to hospital with a child, once we had learned about their perspectives on illness and on their child's vulnerability to illness. We could interpret patterns of usage of preventive health care services, including immunization, in the light of what we learned about how they perceived their job as mothers.

It can be seen that the *focus of the study* was of a particular kind. It was not a detailed study of just one health care topic – like nutrition, or dental care, or use of preventive services. Nor, at the other extreme, was it a study which aimed to cover the whole, very wide, field of child health care. It has the advantage that it was focused and provides sources of comparison across topics. It has the disadvantage that it could not explore in great depth any one topic.

In *method*, too, it was of a specific kind. There were two main approaches. There was some direct questioning. This included some 'closed-end' questions: 'Can you tell me where you were born?' 'Have you taken your child to the clinic in the last six months?' And it included some questions asking mothers to expand on a point: 'Would you say your doctor is a good doctor? ... Why? ... What's good about him/her ... and what, if anything is bad?' The second main approach was to ask mothers to tell the story of recent events – recent illnesses, visits to the doctor, and so on. The first approach directs the interviewee's attention somewhat towards the interviewer's interests. People may reply briefly or at greater length depending on how interesting or important the question seems to them. In giving a reply to such questions of opinion people probably rely on experience, but to some extent they may rely on common opinions of what a good doctor is like and measure their doctor against such opinions. Or they may have an overall view that the doctor is 'good' and then dredge up reasons why this is so to satisfy the interviewer. However, these answers do give some guidance to people's perspectives. The second approach allows people much more freedom to explore and reflect on recent events. As Cornwell (1984) suggests they can turn away from the interview and towards these experiences, and introduce and expand on points that matter to them.

Thus the study used a few structured and many semi-structured questions and also gave mothers the opportunity to describe their views and experiences with very little direction imposed by the interviewer.

What Kind of Status or 'Truth' Does the Information Have?

Commentators on studies based on interviews often cast doubt on the reliability of informants. It is perhaps necessary to comment on this point. Information on topics such as mothers' educational level, length of residence in present housing and so on have been used as variables for analysis, for instance mothers' satisfaction with her health visitor was set against the length of time she said she had known her health visitor. It is assumed that, by and large, mothers gave reasonably accurate information about, for instance, events, times, durations and dates. Possibly some forgot or misremembered, but such cases 'come out in the wash' if there are a reasonable number of cases overall. There are two other reasons for taking mothers' accounts at face value. One is that on many topics, and certainly for this range of topics, there is no better source of information than the child's main caregiver. Secondly, even where there are other sources (such as clinic records) there is no particular reason to believe they are better. Some records are written and others are in the mind but both are subject to error. Indeed a recent study has shown that mothers are sometimes more accurate than medical records (Joffe and Grisso, 1984). However, it should be borne in mind throughout this book that everything said about mothers' circumstances and their health care derives from their accounts. For brevity's sake, the point is not repeated too often.

Much of the information consists of mothers' accounts of their knowledge, their reasons for health practices, their opinions of health services. The data comes from a fairly relaxed interview, as explained above, and we thought mothers told us what they thought rather than what they wanted us to hear. But it was data collected on one occasion, for each mother, and it therefore reflects what each mother thought of saying then, probably in the light of recent events and experiences. Rather than necessarily being true for each mother for all time, this study provides information which gives an account of patterns of beliefs, reasoning and practices that can be discerned when all the mothers' accounts are considered together. It allows one to see whether groups of mothers had distinctive patterns of child health care.

How to Deal with the Information

Mothers' health care of toddlers is territory that has been little explored, so a major aim was to give a broad descriptive account of what we learned about it from the 135 mothers. This work has led to some hypotheses. For instance, it suggests that the work of caring for children's health has some specific characteristics that may help explain parental and professional behaviour. These hypotheses and lines of thought are put forward to stimulate discussion and further research.

The information also allows for analysis by a variety of background factors such as education, housing, income, and by the overarching variable, class. The number of 'cases' – 135 – is sufficient to allow distinctive patterns of care to be distinguished according to such factors. These comparisons were tested for statistical significance using chi squares or rank correlations, depending on the type of variables. Differences between groups of mothers are referred to in this book *only* where they reach statistical significance at the $p < .05$ level or better.[1] But many of the background variables were highly correlated with each other and so it was not appropriate in most cases to go on and try to identify which of, say, income or housing was more important as a factor relating to, say, safety care.

The information collected suggests that the strategies used were useful. It is helpful to consider use of services in the context of health care at home; and to set what people do against what they think important. Needless to say, the work done here points to the need for more work, in greater depth and with other samples. Meanwhile, this study suggests some ideas about how health services can help parents care for their children's health.

Types of Explanation

Finally, it is worth drawing attention to a topic that is important throughout the book. The study offers various types of explanation for differences between groups of mothers.

First, there are mothers' explanations given in answer to direct questions, such as 'Why do you do that?' These are explanations produced, as it were, to order. They may or may not reflect what an individual mother thinks on other occasions, but probably do provide some insight into what reasons are relevant to a group of mothers.

Secondly, there are the explanations one can infer from stories told about, say, a trip to the hospital. A mother might recall, 'I took him to the hospital. I ran all the way with him. He was so hot. He was burning up. He'd never been hot like that before.' This account suggests that the severity and novelty of the symptom and the problem of interpreting it accounted for her journey and for the speed of the journey for medical help. The ordering of the sentences suggests a train of thought.

Thirdly, there are explanations in the form of strong associations between variables. Thus, children having a poor diet tended to live in families with low incomes. In that limited sense, poverty accounts for poor diet, though it does not explain it. Some commentators might argue that poverty is a proxy for fecklessness and that this characteristic provides an explanation for poor diet. In many cases where 'background' variables were set against health care practices and ideas this was as a follow-up to what mothers suggested. Thus among the mothers living in poverty a substantial proportion told us they could not afford good food. In other cases, however, we investigated associations which we thought interesting; thus we set educational level against what mothers said, though no mother suggested this as a relevant factor.

Fourthly, there is broader interpretation by the researcher. Thus consideration of mothers' preventive health care at home led to identification of a set of characteristics of that behaviour. These provided a framework for trying to explain their use of health services.

Fifthly, the values of the researcher critically affect what is studied and what interpretation is given of the findings. Thus it would be possible to study health beliefs and practices without reference to the material circumstances within which mothers rear their children. However, in this study we took the view that the former must be studied and interpreted in the context of the latter.

Given this range of types of explanation, and no doubt there are more, how one interprets and explains findings is a contentious and difficult matter. Interview data of the kind collected in this study cannot be subjected to the sort of analysis that shows what proportion of a finding can be accounted for by a certain variable. What variables one chooses to think important is largely a matter of judgement. In this book both writer and reader have to remain aware of what kinds of explanation are being offered and what kind of weight to put on them.

Note to Chapter 2

1 Where such comparisons are noted the p-value is not quoted. But to point to the strength of the probability the following convention is adopted.

For $p < .05$: the sentence will refer to '*more* mothers ...' or 'mothers are *more likely to* ...'

For $p < .01$: '*many more* mothers ...' or 'mothers are *much more likely to* ...'

For $p < .001$: '*very many more* mothers ...' or 'mothers are *very much more likely to* ...'

A formal report on the study containing more numbers, percentages, tables and significances is lodged with the Economic and Social Research Council (Mayall and Grossmith, 1984).

3

Household Resources for Child Health Care

When a household of two adults is increased by the arrival of a child, two important resource changes take place. Costs go up and income goes down. The child has to be fed, clothed, kept clean and warm – it all costs money; and she has to be supervised constantly. Between them parents provide the care and supervision or pay someone else to do it; if both work, costs of substitute care are high, if one stays at home her or his income is lost. In addition to facing lower income and higher costs, some parents may find that resources that were acceptable before the birth of the child are no longer appropriate. For instance two adults can live well in one or two rooms high off the ground with no lift, no telephone and no car. Caring for a baby in these circumstances is difficult. Indeed parents aim to move into accommodation suitable for child rearing before a child is born, though poorer parents cannot afford to, and under council housing policies may get suitable housing only after the birth of a child, or children (c.f. Ineichen, 1979).

So there are likely to be discrepancies in the resources parents have for health care of their young children, broadly reflecting socio-economic circumstances. All parents want to give their children good care. The question then is, are some of them hindered by their circumstances? And is it reasonable to expect an equal standard of child care from people, no matter what their circumstances?

These questions lie behind the topics addressed in this chapter: the resources households have for health care, and the variations between groups of households in the quality and quantity of resources.

The topics covered here are ones mothers thought affected their health care work or which our analysis showed to be factors that accounted for group differences. Broadly they were housing and the neighbourhood environment; people as a resource for child care; income; and mothers' education. (Perhaps it is worth noting that some factors we initially thought might be explanatory factors did not turn out to be so: mothers' age, religion and whether they did paid work.)

The Study Area and the Housing

First the neighbourhood and the housing. Health care is likely to be critically affected by these, in several respects. Notably, how easy it is to keep children *safe* depends on characteristics of the housing and surrounding streets. How much opportunity parents can give their children for *active play* inside and outside depends on space inside and access to space outside – whether in a garden or a park. Many mothers emphasize *fresh air* as good for health – and the air feels fresher in parks and gardens than in traffic-filled streets. Manoeuvring children, push-chairs and shopping bags out of the home to get to the shops for food – another health care job – can be a stressful chore or a pleasant trip, depending on characteristics of the route: whether there are steps or lifts or a level exit from home to street, whether or not you have to negotiate busy roads to reach the shops.

The area chosen for the study covers about a third of an inner London borough. It measures no more than two miles across in any direction. It is densely populated, with no large green spaces, though there are several large parks just outside the area. There are several wide through roads carrying fast moving heavy traffic in and out of central London, and across the borough. All roads are dangerous for pedestrians, but some seemed to us much more so than others. From our own experience of negotiating the roads on foot and by car, we agreed (without difficulty) on a categorization of roads into 'dangerous' – those with fast heavy traffic – and 'other' roads. In our sample, 39 per cent of the households lived on dangerous roads and 61 per cent on other roads. Most of the mothers went about the borough on foot. Only 24 per cent had use of a car during the week. Bus routes are mainly up and down the borough rather than across it, but distances within our patch were small, so local health services, playgroups and shops and parks were not far on foot.

The borough as a whole shares many of the characteristics of other inner London boroughs.[1] The population has declined in the last decade. It has high rates of poor housing, as measured by overcrowding, and absence of basic amenities. There are high proportions of households headed by lone parents, of households in classes IV and V, of mothers of under-fives in paid work, and of poor people, including disadvantaged groups among ethnic minorities. These characteristics mean that there is acute need for extra resources to meet service needs and to reverse decay and decline. With other inner city boroughs, this one has been classed as a deprived borough, in need of extra resources, under the Inner Urban Areas Act (1978). However, this does not mean that study households were all deprived. In this study we excluded the most needy parts of the borough, as well as the most solidly affluent, in order to get a good class mix.

To say that a borough is deprived does not mean that everyone living there is deprived, on whatever criteria are being used (c.f. Hall and Lawrence, 1981). Like some other inner areas this one has its attractions – it has pleasant neighbourhoods, and it is near to work and the amenities of central London. House prices suggest that competition to live in the borough is high. It attracts some well-to-do people who buy houses and flats, and it also has a proportion of settled people – born and brought up in the area – who may be home owners or, more often, council tenants. For some people the area is home, where they choose to live, though other people – poorly housed in dangerous neighbourhoods – long to leave.

The housing in the area is mostly late Victorian and Edwardian terraced houses, and postwar council flats and houses built on estates. The older houses are semi-detached or terraced, on two or more floors, with gardens. As mothers saw it, the advantages of these houses were that they were spacious, with halls and stairways providing extra play space. They had safe enclosed gardens. But stairways were also safety hazards, as were large, easily accessible windows. Some of the bigger houses had been split into flats and or maisonettes, either as council properties or owner-occupied properties. They had the same sorts of advantages and disadvantages as the houses: good play space but dangerous stairs and windows. The garden was either shared or split lengthways into two long narrow spaces. Either way the household upstairs tended not to use it much, because the children could not easily be supervised. Fifty-eight per cent of the households lived in all or part of an old house.

Most of the rest of the households lived in local authority housing flats on estates, and a few in new (1970s) council houses. Some of this housing provided a pleasant living space: clean, with well-equipped kitchens and safe central heating. The newest estates had been carefully planned so that car routes were separate from pedestrian walkways and sitting out areas. Mothers commented on the relative safety of their journeys across the estate compared to the traffic hazards of older estates.

The two major differences between the older houses and the council properties were in the amount of space available and in the height off the ground. First, the council properties, especially the newest ones, felt cramped – the rooms were small and furniture took up a lot of the space. The few gardens were tiny patches, the size of another small room. So the children did not have much scope for safe active play. Nor could the mother get the child from under her feet for a while. If there was a designated play area outside, it was not enclosed and anyway it was too far away for many toddlers to be happy there on their own. The mother would have to be there too. She could not, as in a house, keep an eye on the children from the window.

Secondly, many of the households lived off the ground floor (67 per cent of the council tenants compared to 8 per cent of the owners) and this restricted the children even more. They had to be stopped from disturbing the people downstairs, and they had to be kept inside the front door because of the dangers of lifts, stairways and balconies. Mothers had the daily problem of manoeuvring children, shopping bags and pushchairs safely up and down the stairs and lifts.

Among the council estates some had multiple disadvantages (in our view). Twenty-two of the households (16 per cent) lived there. These estates had large, high blocks of flats with open-access stone steps leading to open balconies, with the front doors opening off the balcony. Mothers thought this was an outstanding hazard – 23 per cent of all mothers mentioned it – the front door had to be kept locked and bolted to stop the children getting out, and they had to be constantly watched and restrained in case they learned to manipulate the various locking devices. On the balcony the dangers were two-fold: the children could climb up and fall over, or could run along to the stone steps and fall down. There were other hazards too. Because the estates were large, with open access to anyone, mothers did not know, or trust everyone around. These estates were unpopular, so people moved in and out, and mothers were unhappy about some of the households, which they thought socially unacceptable. Fear of hostile or violent people was expressed by a considerable proportion of mothers in classes III, IV and V (16 per cent), most of them living in these flats.

But other characteristics of these estates were dangerous too. They had concreted entrances and parking areas which served for both cars and pedestrians. Even with the child held tightly by the hand, this was dangerous. Some of the estates had no play space for young children, and if they did it was bleak, uninviting, not safely enclosed, and looked dangerous with large-scale equipment (swings, slides) set in concrete. In addition the estates seemed to us (and to mothers) dirty and littered, often with broken glass about. Some had rubbish shutes on each landing opposite the stairs. These are difficult to keep clean and they were often dirty and buzzing with flies. The dirtiness and dangers of the estates led mothers to say they could not foresee a time when their children would be able to play out.

Finally, five of the households were living in homeless family accommodation. This was in large houses or ex-hotels where each family had one room and shared a communal kitchen and bathroom. In some cases meals were also provided communally. Living there might be alright for a few days, but it was obviously very difficult for longer – though some families stay for six months or more. Supervising a child is hard where your kitchen is up a flight of stairs, and shared by others. Inside the room there was virtually no floor space except for corridors between beds, chairs and tables. Keeping dangerous equipment like kettles and irons out of the way was difficult. One child burnt herself on an iron which the mother had stored away under a bed – for safety. Keeping children quiet was a major problem. The households had also been cut off from their own neighbourhood networks – of friends and relatives, and might be far away from their doctors and clinics, so getting help and looking after the children's health was an extra problem. In mitigation, the mothers said they all helped each other and the people running the hostels also provided support and contacts with services.

What Kind of Housing Did the Most and Least Socially Advantaged Families Have?

All but two of the 15 professional households (class I) lived in a whole house. All but one owned their property and had more than one room for each person. Typically they lived in semi-detached Victorian houses on several floors with large rooms, a small front garden and a rectangular patch at the back. All the households had a garden, and had their main living accommodation on the ground floor. In an area where on our rating over half the roads were dangerous, four-fifths of these households had bought a house on a relatively quiet road. For the children all this means that they had plenty of space to run about inside and outside without the likelihood of bumping into things, and they could let off steam in the garden safely. Because parents owned the property and were fairly well off, they could adapt the house as they pleased to make it safe – for instance blocking in bannisters, putting extra doors or locks, laying thick carpets at the bottom of the stairs. Though every mother was worried about road safety at least these children and their parents had a relatively quiet road immediately outside their front door.

The mothers thought that looking after a child's welfare and safety in these circumstances was managable, given the constraints all Londoners face – busy roads, poor transport facilities, dirty parks and roads, pollution. They were all happy with their housing, though 40 per cent would have liked a larger garden. This is not to say that they did not see dangers and intractable safety problems in their housing – for instance large windows and stairs – but they were in general satisfied.

Children in the 26 class IV and V households lived in very different circumstances. Only three lived in a house, and seven had their own garden. Most households had little room for each person; on the crude person:room index, 62 per cent had one or more persons per room. Most (73 per cent) lived above the ground floor. Only one household owned their dwelling. Four were living in homeless family accommodation. Nineteen per cent lived on one of the seven estates which (on our assessment) had multiple disadvantages. For half the households the nearest road was a dangerous, through road.

For these parents keeping the children safe was very difficult. Parents had little money to spend on improvements and devices. Because they did not own the property and might not be there for long they might be unwilling or unable to make it safer. Many of the most dangerous features of the housing could not be altered: the stone steps, the balconies, the rubbish shutes, the play areas, the open access concreted areas. Mothers said they had to keep the children indoors and stop them from active noisy play in case it disturbed the people below. Under these circumstances some of the children were becoming rebellious, wild and difficult to safeguard.

What did these mothers think about their housing from the point of view of their children's safety and welfare? Only a third (31 per cent) were happy. Two-fifths (39 per cent) said there was nothing good about it at all and the rest had many reservations. Many wanted, like parents everywhere, a house and garden for their children. In all, 42 per cent wanted a house or a better flat and 54 per cent more play space – indoors or outdoors. As for roads – every mother was worried about road accidents, but for mothers living on especially busy roads the problem was acute. Every expedition outside the estate meant negotiating a dangerous road.

The comparison between the housing of the socially most advantaged and the most disadvantaged households shows the extreme ends of a continuum from class I through to classes IV and V. Table 3.1 summarizes the picture for each class group. Most households in class II shared the advantages of class I households, though rather more lived in flats without gardens, including a quarter in council accommodation or housing association accommodation. Class III households had similar housing to those in classes IV and V, though more had ground floor flats with gardens.

So the households divided broadly into two main groups according to class. The socially advantaged group owned relatively safe, spacious housing which, within limits, they could improve. The disadvantaged group had more dangerous housing which they were unable to alter and their children had to be restricted in cramped spaces.

Table 3.1 *Households' housing and neighbourhood by father's class (Registrar General)*

	I		II		III		IV, V		
Tenure	N	%	N	%	N	%	N	%	Total N
own	14	93	30	75	6	11	1	4	51
other	1	7	10	25	48	89	25	96	84
Type of housing									
house	13	87	25	63	9	17	3	12	50
other	2	13	15	37	45	83	23	88	85
Garden									
own	15	100	28	70	19	35	5	19	67
shared	0	0	5	13	6	11	3	12	14
none	0	0	7	17	29	54	18	69	54
Floor									
ground	15	100	31	78	21	39	7	27	74
first	0	0	7	18	12	22	6	23	25
second or above	0	0	2	5	21	39	13	50	36
Overcrowding (persons per room)									
under 1	13	87	30	75	21	39	10	39	74
1 or more	2	13	10	25	33	61	16	61	61
(1½ or more)	1	6	0	0	7	13	3	12	(11)
Multiply disadvantaged estate									
No	15	100	38	95	39	72	21	81	113
Yes	0	0	2	5	15	28	5	19	22
Nearest road is dangerous									
No	12	87	31	78	27	50	13	50	83
Yes	3	13	9	22	27	50	13	50	52
No. of mothers	15		40		54		26		135

In order to provide a summary of the households' housing and neighbourhood environment, thinking of it always from the point of view of parents caring for young children's health, we devised an *environmental index*. This took into account whether they lived at ground floor level, whether they lived on one of the multiply disadvantaged estates and whether the nearest road was

Table 3.2 *Environmental index by father's class (Registrar General (%))*

	Environmental Index			
	Good	Average	Poor	N
I	80	20	0	15
II	60	35	5	40
III	22	28	50	54
IV, V	19	23	58	26
N	53	38	44	135

Kendall's Tau C = .48; $p < .001$.
All rows sum to 100%.

'dangerous'. Table 3.2 shows how the households with fathers in high status jobs were also materially advantaged in their housing and neighbourhood, compared to those with fathers in classes III, IV and V.

Income

The notes given above on housing suggest wide disparities in material resources for child health care, according to class. In all, 10 per cent of fathers were unemployed. Most of them had previously worked in class III, IV or V jobs. It was notable that in only one of these households did the mother do paid work.

Non-employment by wives of unemployed men (especially in working class homes) has been documented over the years by the General Household Survey. It has been suggested that the women are unlikely to have marketable skills and that the social security system is a disincentive to the women working, because household benefit will be reduced (OPCS, 1983; Moss, 1976). It also seems that in some households the division of labour does not change when men become unemployed. The woman's job is still housework and child care; the man's to seek paid work.

Of all the mothers, 38 per cent did some paid work, 23 per cent part time and 15 per cent full time (30-plus hours per week); almost all these had only one child. Juggling two children, paid work and pre-school provision is more than most can manage except the very lucky or the very affluent (who can afford nannies and private nurseries). Mothers from classes I and II were very much more likely to do paid work (60 per cent) than those in class III (26 per cent) and those in classes IV and V (19 per cent). Mothers in classes I and II were mostly continuing their careers part time – they could afford to do so because they could pay for care by nannies, in nurseries and at minders out of their salary and still make a reasonable sum. Cheaper forms of care such as play groups do not offer long enough hours to do work for more than an hour or two.

Thus, as for so many of the points in this chapter, one kind of 'good' reinforces or aids another. The women who could command a reasonable salary, living in households with a man in a well-paid professional or management job, were able to arrange their work and substitute child care to suit them, and they made extra money into the bargain. Women in households where men did less well paid, manual work, which also carried a high risk of unemployment, were less well able to afford pre-school care, and so less able to find employment in order to increase the household income.

Not surprisingly, therefore, household income was very closely related to class – high with high and low with low.[2] Only 4 per cent of classes I and II households had a net income of less than £100 per week, compared to 33 per cent of class III and 80 per cent of class IV and V households. Correspondingly, for net incomes over £150 a week the percentages were 67 per cent, 15 per cent and nil.

Telephones and cars

Anyone looking after young children needs easy access to the outside world. Since parents want to give their children 24-hour supervision, they need to be able to run the household, make social contacts, summon help and go for help without leaving the child unattended. In particular, obtaining help from the health services is much easier if you have a phone and a car. It is useful to be able to discuss problems with health visitors and doctors over the telephone, to telephone for a home visit or to arrange a visit to a clinic or surgery. And it is faster, easier and warmer to take a sick child by car to consult health professionals. One mother whose children both developed high temperatures late at night explained how a phone call had helped:

She just burned up and became delirious. I phoned the doctor and he advised Calpol and I was reassured enough to try what he suggested and it worked. They both had coughs (aged 35 and 5 months). With the baby he suggested wrapping her up in a blanket and covering her – all the things you would do anyway, but he said try and calm down yourself, take some aspirin for yourself first, so I did all that, and just the fact, talking to him, calmed me down enough to deal with it. And I gave Sandra some Calpol and we all eventually went to sleep. It was about 11 o'clock at night, a Friday night – things often happen on a Friday night.

Another mother who had no telephone and no car explained how she cared for her ill child. She felt she had to take risks with her child's health. (She had taken her son, 21 months, to doctor that day with a high temperature. He had a throat swab taken.)

That night he was quite ill. I was quite worried about him. It's awkward not being on the phone. My husband was at work. I just virtually stayed by his bed all night – he wanted sponging down and little sips of orange squash now and then. He was asleep but he kept moaning and whimpering in his sleep. He was quite sort of distressed. I didn't take his temperature again, because I could feel he was quite hot. I gave him the Calpol that evening before I tried to settle him down. In the morning his temperature seemed to have come down, but he was still a bit hot. Lunchtime he had a little sleep. When he woke he was sticky, it had broken, he'd sort of sweated it all out in his sleep. So by three in the afternoon he was more or less better. If I'd had a phone I might have called the doctor in to have a look, because as I say I had to prop a pillow underneath him, under the mattress, to raise it because his breathing was a bit difficult, he was really panting, a little bit wheezy.

Obviously, ownership of these useful telephones and cars depends on affluence, and all the households in class I had phones and all but one a car. Ownership declined along the class continuum; only 38 per cent of households in classes IV and V had phones and 46 per cent had a car.

Household's ownership of a car does not necessarily mean that the parent caring for the child has the use of it. In our 135 households 65 per cent had a car but only 24 per cent of mothers had the use of the car on weekdays (and knew how to drive). Most of these (78 per cent) lived in class I and II households, where nearly half the mothers had use of the car – 45 per cent compared to only 7 per cent of mothers in the other class groups.

Table 3.3 *Proportion of households owning a car and a phone, by father's class*

| Household has: | Father's class | | | | No. of households |
	I	II	III	IV, V	
Own car	93	75	59	46	88 (65%)
Own phone	100	93	70	38	100 (74%)
No. of households	15	40	54	26	135

People as a Resource

Numbers of adults in the household

All the children in this study lived in two-parent households, and in almost all cases (93 per cent) there were no other people in the household. Most of the 135 mothers (68 per cent) had just the one child – the focus child, aged 18–36 months. The rest had a second child, of whom three-quarters were under 1 year old. So on paper there were two adults to care for one or two children.

However, mothers' accounts show that in practice most mothers did most of the caring. Most of the fathers saw their children for no longer than an hour or two at the beginning or end of the day, though 22 per cent, equally from all class groups, were present and 'helped' or 'shared' the care or 'took over' at other times – at mid-day, in the early evening, if they worked part time or on shifts, or if they were unemployed (10 per cent of fathers). Some fathers worked very long hours, and in a few cases they spent periods of time living and working away from the home. In addition mothers' stories revealed recent temporary separations where parents had had a row, and three fathers had been in prison in the last year. All in all, the accounts of child care discussed in the following chapters consistently show that traditional patterns were operating. Most fathers were not there during the day or did not do the caring. One example will serve here to point this up: of 71 children taken to the GP in the last three months, 69 went with their mother.

Still, fathers were an important resource for health care. In an emergency they took time off work and got the child to hospital, or took over shopping or child care if the mother was ill. In some cases mothers (and fathers, if present) told us they shared child care perhaps not equally, but each took responsibilities for some jobs or for some parts of the day; some decisions were made jointly.

Caring for young children's health demands not only the presence of adults, but the adults' *good health*. Relationships between parental and child health is a neglected and important topic – one that is the focus of a current Thomas Coram Research Unit study. Meanwhile, this study throws some light on it (see Chapter 8). Mothers' accounts of their care of their children in the last three months show that in 33 per cent of households adult ill health had posed problems. Mainly, mothers had been ill with pregnancy or recent childbirth and some fathers had been ill too. Reports of adult ill health as it affected care of the child did not vary by class.

Adult ill health caused problems for parents caring for their ill children, but it could also cause more ill health generally in the household. Ill parents found it difficult to care for an ill child; mothers found it harder to care for a sick man and a sick child. Children and adults caught illness from each other, and ill children were distressed and disturbed when their mother or father became ill, so an ill parent would be constrained both by her own illness and by the child's reaction in caring for that child.

Thus, resources varied between households in terms of number of adults carrying out health care work and their own health status. There were no clear differences by class. In general it seemed that most mothers did most of the caring. In about a third of the households adult ill health caused problems recently in caring for ill children.

Relatives and friends

People from outside the households can also help parents with health care: relatives and friends; and people who take over or share the care – minders, nannies, playgroup leaders and nursery staff. Mothers talk to people about their children in order to tell their own stories, to exchange notes, to ask advice, to learn from others' experiences, and in a general way to gain and give each other support. Relatives and friends can help mothers decide what action to take for a sick child and whether to consult a professional.

> I phoned my friend, Jean, not particularly for advice, just to talk about it (respiratory condition). She's got two children, so she's seen it all. I find her a very down-to-earth person, very sensible.

> I mentioned it to my mother (earache) and she just said if he complains again or starts crying take him to the doctor, 'cos you shouldn't poke around yourself.

> I talked to various friends – their children had had the same thing (diarrhoea) and had taken them to the doctor and got nowhere. All they (doctors) say is, here's some antibiotics. And I discussed it with my husband and we agreed to wait and see.

Among the 135 mothers, three-quarters felt they had enough people to talk with about their children's health and welfare, but a substantial minority (24 per cent) did not. Mothers seemed to need to see at least one person (apart from the father) almost every day, and three or four people a week, if they were to feel satisfied with the level of social support they had. Apart from the father, who acted as confidant for 86 per cent of mothers, their own mother was the main confidante (for 53 per cent of mothers).

There was a broad class divide on satisfaction with social support. Mothers in classes I and II were more likely to be satisfied than other mothers (85 per cent against 69 per cent). Though there are no totally clear-cut explanations in the findings for this, some aspects of the households' circumstances suggest reasons. First of all, parents in classes I and II were more likely to have settled into their present housing before their first child was born, and they were very much less likely to have moved house in the last year (7 per cent compared to 13 per cent in class III and 27 per cent in classes IV and V). Secondly, as already noted, there was a decrease along the class continuum in ownership of phones and cars. So most mothers in classes I and II had had time to establish good friendships and were able to keep in touch with other friends and with relatives by phone and to visit by car. In classes III, IV and V there were some mothers (36 per cent) who had lived all their lives in the borough and had frequent supportive contacts with relatives – especially with mothers and sisters. But other mothers had had contacts with relatives and friends disrupted by moving house and fewer had telephones and cars which would have helped them to keep in touch.

Playgroup leaders, minders and others

Playgroup leaders, minders, nursery staff and nannies help mothers care for their children's health in important ways. Some politicians and policy-makers may see pre-school provision as a matter for private decisions and private payment. In practice it can be critically important for parents, especially for mothers. For a start, it may enable them to do paid work, and so provide extra household income, or the sole household income. In a poor household the mothers' earned income may make all the difference between stretched resources and a reasonable standard of living. Later chapters show that some mothers felt unable to give their children all they needed for good health, because of low income. For some mothers holding onto the job after childbirth is essential if they intend to work in the foreseeable future for in these days of high unemployment women may not be able to break back into a job or into a career once they leave. Women's life-time earnings chances are affected by these gaps in employment. In addition the satisfaction of working is important to many mothers; they are not likely to give their children good care if they are bored, frustrated and miserable at home. Pre-school provision also gives mothers a break. It is not frivolous for mothers to want a break; many need one, to relax, to get the strength together to care for the child, to talk with friends without children's interruptions, as well as to do shopping and household jobs. Then they can take up child care again refreshed.

People who provide substitute care are also a source of help and support for mothers and can give useful perspectives on the child's health or development. For instance mothers referred to the local knowledge of minders, or the opinions of nursery staff.

> My childminder said all the children round here had it (a chesty cough). She thought it was worth getting something from the chemist, or going to the doctor.
>
> His nursery teacher said she thought he was slightly deaf, and we might want to check it with the doctor.

But in Britain pre-school provision is scarce and expensive for parents. It is especially so for the under-threes, for whom most places are in the private sector, at minders or nurseries. The really well-to-do can hire nannies and au pairs. State nursery schools are free and playgroups fairly cheap but most take children only at three, and for two or three hours – so they do not give mothers much of a break, or free time for paid work.

Half the focus children (54 per cent) spent some time with caregivers other than their parents, mostly at playgroups, or with neighbours, friends and minders. More of the older than of the younger children did so. Most of this substitute care was part-time; only 20 per cent of the 135 children spent 20 hours or more a week with other caregivers. Children from classes I and II were very much more likely to have some substitute care (78 per cent) than those in class III (46 per cent) and especially compared to those in classes IV and V (31 per cent) and this was irrespective of whether the mother did paid work. Why parents used pre-school provision was not a topic of this study, but class I and II mothers were better able to afford it and some used it at least partly so they could do paid work. Other studies suggest that middle class mothers are better at cornering this scarce resource (e.g. Hughes *et al.*, 1980). High mobility is also a barrier to using pre-school care; it takes time to find somewhere or someone and there is no point in starting a child off with a stranger if you are likely to be moving out of the area. And if you live in very poor housing and under a good deal of stress, taking a child to playgroup for a couple of hours may be more than you feel you can manage.

Mother's education

Mothers care for their children's health partly in the light of their perceptions of what constitutes good care. They bring to the job their own experiences as children and adults, the knowledge passed on by their parents, what they learn on the job in discussion with the child's father and with relatives and friends, and what they learn from teachers and health professionals. Among these kinds of knowledge, mother's access to the sorts of knowledge health professionals would like us to have and put into practice was important in this study. One crude indicator of this access is mother's educational level.

People's chances of good education are closely tied to their home backgrounds. Children from working class backgrounds, compared to other children, still have poor chances of getting external examination qualifications. Thus for 1981/82, 68 per cent of people aged 25–49 whose fathers were in class V had no qualifications, compared to 7 per cent of people from class I

Table 3.4 *Father's occupational class (Registrar General) by mother's education*

Mother's education	I	II	IIINM	IIIM	IV, V	N
Group A	14	37	5	17	4	77
Group B	1	3	4	28	22	58
N	15	40	9	45	26	135

Group A = minimum 'O' levels (including training for professional work).
Group B = maximum CSEs (including training for IIINM or IIIM work).

backgrounds. Similarly, only 2 per cent of them went on to get a degree compared to 31 per cent of people from class I backgrounds. There was also a sex difference. Among children with fathers in manual occupations, particularly few girls went on to get degrees, and many had no qualifications, compared to boys. The sex differences were less pronounced, though still clear, in children from non-manual backgrounds (OPCS, 1984, ch. 7, especially Table 7.5). It is not appropriate here to consider in detail why this class difference persists in the face of 'free' and 'open-access' secondary education. But the class differences in children's educational chances are gross and persistent and must reflect differences in material advantage between class groups. Leaving aside parents' hopes for their children and their different treatment of boys and girls, teachers' expectations of children and variations between schools as possible explanatory factors, at the base-line it is clear that for parents to keep children in education after the minimum leaving age (16) means allocating substantial resources for maintenance and in some cases fees, as well as foregoing the child's earnings. It is known that many children leave school at the Easter before public exams in order to contribute to household income. Overall, it is clear that education is a material good: children get it if their homes are materially advantaged.

By and large women with certain class backgrounds and the education to match tend to set up homes with men from similar backgrounds (Leete and Fox, 1977). In this study mother's educational level was closely related to the father's and to the father's class (Registrar General). For those who want more detail, it is set out in the Appendix, but the essential points are given briefly here.

For some purposes in this study mother's educational level is used as a variable on its own to see whether it was related to differences in kinds of health belief and health practice. But we also thought it might be useful to have an indicator that took into account both father's class and mother's education. This would serve to point to a composite of kinds of advantage – material, social and educational. Using the findings shown in Table 3.4, we devised a 'Mother's Class', which recognized the close relationship between father's class and mother's education at both ends of the class continuum and the variation in class III. We subdivided the 54 class III households into two. First, those where the father was in a III non-manual job or the mother had 'O' levels: this gave 26 households, called class IIIa. Second, those where the father was in III manual work and the mother had no training, or qualifications above CSE: this gave 28 households, called IIIb. For the purposes of this study, Mother's Class was often a good discriminator, showing that there were broad divisions between mothers in classes, I, II and sometimes IIIa, and those in classes IIIb, IV and V.

As we shall show, mother's education was a resource for health care, in the sense that high levels of education appeared to give mothers access to certain sorts of health knowledge – the messages that health professionals beam at parents. This is not to say that those messages will be implemented nor, if they are, that such practices will necessarily give children better chances of health. Nor does the fact of a relationship between education and types of knowledge or information explain the mechanisms of the relationship. But it was the case that highly-educated mothers referred to more items of knowledge that fitted with health education messages as compared with other mothers. And clearly mothers who know what health professionals recommend have an advantage in deciding how to care for their children and in relating to professionals.

Resources and Health Care

In this chapter some important resources for the health care of young children have been considered: housing, the neighbourhood, income, amenities, people and their health, mother's education. For this sample of households it was clear that the sorts of advantages people think of when they divide households by class held good. Those at the top of the class continuum tended to have all the advantages: adequate income, housing and neighbourhoods, help with child care, satisfaction with social support, high levels of education. Some of those at the bottom of the continuum had most of the corresponding disadvantages.

It is worth noting that on the whole social policy in this country does not recognize the specific needs of households with young children for extra or different resources. There is no coordinated policy to ensure that parents have adequate resources to rear their children. Local authorities do take responsibility for housing people with children, though in cities the housing they have provided has, until recently, been in flats, off the ground — which most parents consider unsuitable for child rearing. And there is child benefit, paid in cash to mothers. But the lobby for this has never been powerful enough to keep the rate in line with the cost of living and it has never been more than a welcome but minor contribution to the costs of children. While health services for all children and education services from five years are provided free on a universal basis, the health costs of children are not otherwise catered for by social policies. In general it is assumed that parents bear the costs of children themselves out of their wages, and this includes, for under-fives, the costs of substitute care. Yet while the idea of the man's wage as a family wage still holds sway, for instance in negotiations by trades unions, it is known that for many households with children, one wage is insufficient to keep the people out of poverty. Poverty is increasing among two-parent households (McNay and Pond, 1980). But no help in the form of adequate, subsidized pre-school care is promoted by government departments to enable parents to work to raise their standard of living to reasonable levels.

The data set out in this chapter point out the obvious: at the 'lower' end of the occupational class continuum households tend to be poorly resourced in more than one respect. Those in poor housing also have no telephones, no cars, poor education, poor access to pre-school care. At the root of their disadvantage and deprivation is poverty. If a goal of social policy is to produce a healthy population, what are the appropriate measures? It is interesting to look back at measures developed over the course of this century to combat child ill health and to see where we stand now. In the early years of the century, the first intervention was the provision of free school meals to five year olds. Then baby clinics were provided in order to intervene further back in the life-cycle – through the first five years. Later still, recognition was given to the likelihood that unhealthy mothers might bear unhealthy babies. The provision of a free health service has, among other factors, served to improve mothers' health. Now social policy-makers must look to the underlying causes of inequalities in ill health – to the material circumstances in which children are reared.

For professionals dealing with parents and their young children, the difficult task is to offer a useful service to people suffering resource deprivation. In general, baby books and health education literature give little recognition to variations in household resources and how these affect health care work. Health visitors and social workers tend to be aware of interactions of resources with practices, because they visit homes. Doctors may be less well aware of parents' difficulties. On this a recent proposal that GPs improve their knowledge by home visiting is welcome (RCGP, 1982).

The circumstances in which some parents rear their children force the question whether these parents can be expected to give them good care. Does there come a point where material conditions make good parenting impossible? (For instance, Douglas and Blomfield (1958) found that those mothers rated 'inefficient' by health visitors were likely to be living in poor housing, to have many children and to be in poor health.) It is now widely accepted that the physical and social conditions of some estates are unsuitable for child rearing. Homeless family hostels are so too, and evidence of their ill effects on health and health care is urgently needed.

In the next chapter safety care, especially as it relates to housing conditions, is discussed.

Notes to Chapter 3

1 These data derive from the GLC's Social Review of Greater London (1980), 1971 and 1981 Census data, the National Dwelling and Housing Survey (Department of the Environment, 1979) and the National Classification of Residential Neighbourhoods (Webber, 1977).
2 Establishing exact household income is a lengthy task. We aimed for a broad guide to poverty and relative affluence. We asked mothers to indicate net household income (after tax, but including benefits), using a card showing broad income bands.

SECTION B

Preventive Care at Home

4

Safety Care

Introduction

In Chapter 3 the question was raised whether some parents have such poor resources that they *cannot* give their children good care. This chapter considers one crucial kind of care – safety care – in the context of households' housing conditions. As far as mothers are concerned, how well they can ensure their children's safety depends crucially on characteristics of their housing and the neighbourhood environment.

What mothers said about their problems in safeguarding their children provides graphic illustration and explanation of the harsh statistics on accidents. Accidents are the commonest cause of death to children aged 1–14 years. For the age group 1–4 years, 22 per cent (258) of deaths in 1979 were from accidents, the main ones being road accidents, and deaths from fires and drowning. Children from class V households are much more likely to die from accidents than those in class I: 5 to 7 times more likely for road accidents, and even more for deaths from fires, falls and drowning. Boys are more likely than girls to die from accidents in every occupational class except I – which suggests that most parents (except those in class I) socialize boys and girls differently. Deaths are the tip of the accident iceberg. Many children go to Accident and Emergency Departments for accidents – two million children (aged 1–14) in 1979 and one million to GPs. Below this layer are many more accidents, serious and relatively trivial, but mostly distressing – the accidents that are not seen by doctors and do not figure in the statistics.

As has been shown, the households had widely varying

physical environments. Broadly, class I and II households lived in their own house or flat with a garden, on a quiet residential road. Households in classes III, IV and V lived in council flats, mostly off the ground, on estates, many opening onto dangerous through roads. The worst-off households, almost all from classes III, IV and V, lived on estates with multiple disadvantages (22) or in one room in homeless family accommodation (5). Our environmental index summed up the quality of the housing and neighbourhood for child rearing: most class I and II households had a good environment (65 per cent compared to 21 per cent in class III, IV and V households) and very few indeed had a poor one (4 per cent compared to 52 per cent).

Active Children in Poor Housing – a Recipe for Accidents?

It is difficult to describe adequately the intensity and scale of many mothers' dissatisfaction with their housing as an environment for child rearing. To quote some figures: 36 per cent of mothers in classes III, IV and V said there was nothing good at all about their housing (by comparison with 5 per cent in classes I and II). Here three of these unhappy mothers describe the problems. They all lived in the worst estates, above ground floor level.

> There's always risk in the home, mainly for his size. He could bang the window and push the glass. Or he could fall through the glass. It's a sash – we can't change it. He can climb up on the sofa to the window. The flat's too restricted – he's no room to play and he loves climbing. And if there was a fire how would we get out? It worries me terribly. My Nan was in a fire, she was very badly burned. I try to keep him out of the kitchen while I'm cooking, because he can reach up to things. But if I shut him out I can't see what he's up to. My main worry with him would be climbing and drinking disinfectant, if my back was turned. And outside – he – if he escaped – he can't open the front door yet, but there's the stone steps up to the balcony. It's run-down here. The air's not clean, it's a bad environment. There's flies in the rubbish shute. If you go down and open the shute all the rubbish falls out – it's horrible.
>
> We wouldn't have half the trouble we do have if he could get out (into a garden). When we're over my parents he's out in the garden from dawn to dusk. He's safe there, and he's much less wild when he is inside.

We've got half a dozen different locks and bolts on the door. We have to keep putting them higher up. She's desperate to get out, and you have to watch her all the time, cos she's trying to get out. She could run along the balcony and fall down the steps, and there's cars down there.

This next mother is in a new council flat (2nd floor) on an estate. Their front door opens onto a small open landing with low rail and open stone steps.

In a small flat you're a bit confined. So you tend to get in each other's way as well as his (child's) way. So I suppose that makes us safety conscious. I'm going to put a bolt on the front door so he can't get out. At the moment he can't open the door. He's too confined. He's not getting enough exercise. It'll be worse when he's older. I won't be able to let him run around outside because it's a rough area, and the people – it's like any council estate. The windows are very bad. They're low down and they've got loose handles – he'll soon be able to open them. He can reach up to them now. I have to keep the windows shut – it's a problem in these small rooms. It gets very hot. I have to watch him all the time. Keep telling him – it's wrong, mustn't do that. If you tell him he will stay away – like the TV and the video. He never touches it. We've told him no and he obeys. Really I think they have to be disciplined.

These mothers, like many others, were drawing attention both to how the physical environment restricted their children's activity and to the restrictions they as parents had to impose on the children.

The children's high level of activity and behavioural characteristics were seen as normal for their age, but some characteristics were seen as particularly likely to lead to accidents. Mothers thought their children were likely to have accidents because they were clumsy, adventurous, investigative, defiant or just plain accident-prone. Thirty-six per cent of mothers thought their children had two or more of these potentially dangerous characteristics. The proportion rose steadily from 26 per cent in class I to 46 per cent in classes IIIb, IV and V. In particular they thought their children were clumsy and defiant. And where the children were under two, mothers in classes III, IV and V were more likely than the rest to think their children had more potentially dangerous characteristics. Mothers in classes III, IV and V were very much more likely than other mothers to think their *boys* were at risk (54 per cent as against 13 per cent). For girls there was no class difference.

What do these findings mean? Possibly mothers in different social groups expect different things for their young children; perhaps those in the manual working classes think children should not be clumsy and so make much of it, if they are. But this would not explain the sex differences. Here it seems likely (as Black, 1980, suggests) that working-class boys are brought up differently from the girls, encouraged to be active, boisterous, daring, and this may account for their having more fatal accidents than girls, and more accidents (twice as many) as their peers in class I. Research evidence suggests that parents do socialize their children differently, by sex (McGuire, 1983). A probable complementary reason why some children in classes III, IV and V were seen as having potentially dangerous characteristics, and from a younger age, is that they lived in circumstances which provoked certain kinds of behaviour. If family life is crammed into a small flat, especially if it is high off the ground, then the children will constantly have to be restrained, rebuked and contradicted, and so they may become rebellious, and prone to dash off and try the impossible or the dangerous. Children may seem clumsy because in a crowded flat they bang into furniture and break things. So their mothers may define them as defiant and clumsy children. This was in fact the case. More of those mothers in classes III, IV and V thought their children had two or more potentially dangerous characteristics if they lived on the multiply disadvantaged estates than if they lived elsewhere (55 per cent as against 40 per cent), and more of them thought so if they lived on the second floor or above.

These data are not conclusive, but they do suggest that whatever the mechanisms at work, mothers in classes III, IV and V had more worries than other mothers about their children's propensity to accidents. This hypothesis is supported by data giving the other side of the picture. Mothers in classes I and II were much more likely than other mothers to think their children had one or more *safe* characteristics. The characteristics mothers most often referred to were being cautious and being well coordinated. There was no difference between mothers according to the child's age or sex.

> She's very cautious about climbing. She doesn't rush into things. She takes her time, or she asks for your help.
>
> He knows to do things so he's safe. He says 'careful'. Climbing – he doesn't put his feet, his hands so he'll fall.

Keeping Them Healthy as Well as Safe – an Impossible Task?

What the mothers quoted above said about safety care also tells us their ideas about normal healthy behaviour in young children. Children need to play actively, to run and climb, to investigate and explore. These behaviours help children to learn and to grow strong, but they are dangerous when the children live in cramped housing. So for the mothers, keeping them safe meant restricting normal healthy behaviours by means of physical barriers and by prohibitions. It also meant constant vigilance, constant awareness of the child's abilities and interests, and the flexibility to implement a variety of strategies to safeguard the child from her physical environment.

> Plugs – he's a monster for plugs, I have to watch him all the time. And windows – he climbs up on the tumble drier, he could get out from there. We've put screw locks on the windows. I never leave him on his own. There's so many things. You have to keep your eye on such a lot of things. You never go to answer the phone and leave the iron on, or a saucepan on the stove. It just comes automatically to think about that.

> He keeps on going up the stairs. He can climb over the gate (safety gate). I keep bringing him down, and I smack his bottom to try to keep him off. It's an open tread staircase. He could break his arms and his legs if he fell. Very dangerous. He has no idea of danger at all. He doesn't know any fear. He'll try anything. He just doesn't know, he doesn't think about it. He just explores.

But though mothers may do what they think appropriate, children surprise them with newly learned abilities, and they move so fast that they are into danger before you know it:

> Once she went into the kitchen. Why, I couldn't believe it. I was there too, so was her Dad. And she opened one of the cupboard doors – which I didn't know she could do at the time, and she got some disinfectant. And what did she do? I don't know how she did it. But she opened the top and drank some. I couldn't believe it because I put those tops on very well. But she only drank a little. The first thing I did was – I read the directions on the back and it said, keep away from children, but it wouldn't poison children! And she wasn't sick or anything. And since then I've put them higher up.

This mother recalled the incident because the child had demonstrated new, unknown abilities and because the parents, with her in a small room, missed what was happening. She was amazed and in a sense delighted at the new skills her child was developing; yet these very skills led the child into danger. Like other mothers, she thought a healthy child was one who was active and investigative.

So safety care involved mothers in a balancing act between two kinds of health care: encouraging, facilitating or allowing active investigative behaviour; and preventing injury. Getting the balance right was the daily problem the mothers faced. Here is another mother explaining the many skills her child was learning and the safety problems they caused:

> He's more vulnerable to danger now, because he's quicker and more inquisitive. He'll try to take the TV and radio to bits ... And he'll run, and he takes some catching now. The other day he ran away along the pavement ... He's terrible – he'll take the plugs and go into the sockets ... he climbs into the bath ... he climbs up to the window. I've had to take all the chairs out of the kitchen so he can't climb up and reach things. But he can turn on the gas now. He swings on the sofa – on the back; he could fall off.

Strategies for Keeping Children Safe

Almost every mother thought keeping her child safe was a problem and did a lot about it. Their spontaneous comments were mainly about safety at home, since there was more they could do there: the environment was more controllable. But every mother talked spontaneously too about road dangers and the precautions they took. The topics we asked about specifically, in order to get information from all mothers, were falls, burns and scalds, poisoning, drowning, and electrical accidents. We asked mothers whether they thought there was a risk and whether they did anything about it. Almost every mother took some kind of action about each of the topics we mentioned, and these actions fell into three broad kinds: reliance on the child, supervision and preventive action. These are described in turn, but first a note about circumstances where mothers took *no* action.

No safety action

Virtually all mothers took action against burns and scalds (all but 3) and against poisoning (all but 5). Some took no action against water accidents (28) or electrical dangers (21) because they thought there was no risk. There were no class differences on this, but two important class differences did emerge.

The first was that some mothers felt powerless to make the accommodation safe for the child. They lacked control of the housing. A third of mothers in classes III, IV and V (33 per cent) compared to 11 per cent of other mothers identified aspects of their housing which constituted a danger of falling or bruising to their children but which they could not alter. They were renting property which had unalterable structural dangers: badly placed doors, sharp edges to walls, windows that could not be made child-proof, steep stairs, open-tread stairs, balconies leading to open-access steps. The number of unalterable and dangerous features of their housing mentioned by mothers was very strongly class-related.

The second class difference was on the matter of learning from experience. Mothers in classes I and II were very much more likely than other mothers to think children should run a few risks in order to learn by trial and error, as regards falls and minor burns (33 per cent as against 11 per cent).

> We've never had a stairgate for him. I'd rather he had a few tumbles and learned how to manage the stairs. Then he'll be safe on them.
>
> If you just let them go and run and find out for themselves they will have accidents. I'm not frightened of her having accidents – she has had accidents.
>
> She likes to be with me in the kitchen when I'm doing the cooking and she sits up at the table and the cooker's next to the table and she's never ever attempted to touch a pan or anything that's cooking. Occasionally she's touched a pan and she's had a tiny burn on her finger.

It could be that these mothers had particular theories about child rearing, but mothers are practical people – they would not put a theory into practice if it jeopardized their child's safety. The important distinction here must be that class I and II mothers knew from experience that their housing was sufficiently safe for the children to come to no serious harm – unlike the other mothers, who, as we have seen, thought their children ran very grave risks at home and on the estate, and felt they had to do all in their power to safeguard them.

Reliance on the child

Some mothers felt they could begin to rely on their children, to some extent, to avoid danger, particularly as regards falls and burns. But almost all of these also supervised their children or carried out preventive action or both. They were cautious. For instance, on poisoning: 'He knows about that. We show him a bleach bottle and he says – "dangerous". But I keep all that high up anyway.' And another, on burns:

> There's always a danger with a child this age that doesn't understand. He knows not to touch certain things – he knows the kettle is burny, as we say. He knows the central heating vents are hot – not to touch. He doesn't come near the cooker. He won't come near. He tells *me* now. He picks things up quite fast. I think he knows, but God forbid I should say that and he burn himself this evening.

Few mothers *only* relied on the child: 12 as to avoiding drowning, 9 as to falls, 8 as to burns and electricity and 2 as to poisoning. One mother said about kitchen cleaners: 'She's never really got all the stuff out of the cupboards. And now she knows what they're all for. They're in a cupboard under the sink.' Another said, about drowning: 'She's fine in the bath. She wouldn't put her head under water. I can leave her there to play.'

So mothers observed their children in action and made a decision when to trust them. To an outsider it may seem that some decisions to rely on the children are a bit premature and may be risky. Altogether 22 per cent of the mothers, equally from all classes, relied solely on the child to avoid danger from one or more risk. Few mothers placed any reliance on the child's knowledge of poisoning (12 per cent) or drowning (20 per cent) or electricity (27 per cent). Rather more relied on the child not to fall (38 per cent) or burn herself (47 per cent).

There was no significant class difference in the proportions of mothers who relied on the child to stay safe in connection with each risk; nor according to the age of the child – although rather more mothers of children at the top of the age range relied on them. There were two groups of mothers who we thought might rely more on their children's sense and knowledge: those who were employed full time (30 hours or more) (16 per cent), and those who had two children (32 per cent). Both these groups – which did not overlap – might ascribe to their children a high level of reliability. But this was not so. There was no relationship between working full time or having a second child and the mothers' views. This holds true as well for supervision and preventive action.

Supervision

Most of the mothers spent their days with the children. This does not mean they were in the presence of their children all the time. Most thought it was safe to leave their children in some rooms of the house or flat for a few minutes, either anywhere (30 per cent) or anywhere but the kitchen and bathroom (56 per cent) – which many viewed as the most dangerous rooms. A small proportion (14 per cent) also said they sometimes left the child in the house alone, usually in bed, while they dashed round to the nearest shop or to the telephone. There was no difference between groups of mothers by class or by the child's age on any of this.

We included under 'supervision' both monitoring and teaching. That is, we included mothers' statements about keeping an eye, or an ear on children, removing them from danger, warning them of it and explaining to them why it was dangerous. All mothers monitor their children's activities in these ways – or at least if there are exceptions, we do not think we encountered them. It is such a central and obvious part of what mothers do when they are with their children, that they may not always be

Table 4.1 *Proportion of mothers using various strategies to safeguard their children against certain risks*

Strategy	Falls	Burns/ Scalds	Poisoning	Drowning	Electricity	Roads
None/no risk	11	2	4	21	17	0
Supervision	23	16	2	44	10	45
Reliance	7	6	2	10	7	0
Prevention	15	17	72	7	32	18
Sup. + rel.	13	10	1	7	9	16
Sup. + prev.	14	17	7	10	14	20
Prev. + rel.	12	16	9	1	7	1
All three	6	15	3	2	4	1

All columns sum to 100%. Number of mothers = 135.

aware that they are doing it or mention it in discussion of accident prevention. Of the three strategies we were interested in – reliance, supervision and prevention – this was the one where we got least detail. It seems likely that where mothers thought their preventive actions were adequate they would stress these rather than their own supervisory actions. So the most interesting data on supervision is not that where it was combined with reliance on prevention, but where the mother said that was *all* she did to keep the child safe.

Table 4.1 shows that mothers thought that preventing poisoning was not a matter for supervision alone, whereas nearly half the mothers used it as their sole strategy against drowning and road dangers. Different dangers demand different actions. Though you may help to prevent drowning by, say, putting a rubber mat in the bath, probably the best way is by being with the child. It also seemed that drowning was low in the hierarchy of mothers' fears, since a fifth did nothing about it. On the other hand, poisoning ranked high as a fear, and prevention was the principal strategy. There were no differences on supervision alone, or in conjunction with other measures by class or by the age of the child.

There was a small group of mothers (10) who relied on supervision much more than other mothers did, as the only strategy against three or more types of risk. One of these mothers talked as follows about how she cared for her child:

On burns: There's only a risk if he drags his chair in the kitchen. But he's very rarely on his own in the kitchen.

On poisoning: He can open the cupboard under the sink. But there's always someone with him.

On drowning: There's no problem here, because he's never on his own in the bath.

On electricity: He'll try to plug something in. But there's no danger, because he's not on his own in the room.

On falls: You can't prevent them. Just be there when they fall.

Another said of poisoning risks: 'I wouldn't be that heedless. I wouldn't let her take something.'

These few mothers' comments were worrying because it seemed they thought their own responsible behaviour was enough on its own to keep the child safe. The evidence from other mothers suggests that preventive action was important too.

Preventive action

Under this heading we included physical barriers, restraints and devices, such as gates, fireguards, locks and bolts, mats to soften falls, harnesses in push-chairs and cars.

We collected two kinds of information: first, we asked mothers what they had done about risks (falls, burns, poisoning, drowning, electricity, roads) and secondly, we filled out with the mother a check list of common safety devices. So we got data about individual strategies to beat risks and about more conventional safeguards.

Whether mothers carry out preventive action depends on the risk – it may be less crucial than supervision against drowning, but very important against poisoning and burns, along with supervision. There was general agreement among groups of mothers on these distinctions, and there were no class differences between them as to whether they took preventive action against each of the risks we listed. Preventive action was high for poisoning (90 per cent), burns (65 per cent) and electric shocks (57 per cent), fairly high for falls (47 per cent) and road accidents (40 per cent) and lower for drowning (20 per cent). For road accidents and drowning supervision was all important.

However, factors related to class did affect preventive action. First, as we noted earlier, some mothers were unable to take all the action they thought appropriate against falls. They took some action, but the property in which they lived had structural dangers which they could not alter.

Secondly, the type of preventive action taken differed according to class. There are several ways of preventing any one type of accident, and not all include conventional (perhaps expensive) equipment. For instance, some mothers barred access to electrical sockets with heavy furniture, or they moved sockets. Others bought socket covers – which some children learned to prise off. Mothers might prevent burns from the cooker by turning pan handles in, when the expensive precaution would be a cooker guard, or a gate fixed across the kitchen doorway. Burns might be prevented by never leaving cigarettes or matches around, but not all mothers prevented burns from the fire by installing a fireguard. There were significant class differences in ownership of bought safety devices: socket covers, cooker guards or gates across the doorway, fireguards and car seats. In each case there was a decrease in ownership along the continuum from class I to classes IV and V. It is likely that these class differences have to do with *income*. Households with less than £100 a week, compared to the rest, had fewer cooker safeguards, socket covers, gates and car seats.[1] Given the number of 'cases' it was not possible to analyse the data for income controlled for social class (they were very highly correlated); nor, similarly, for income controlled by tenure. Perhaps there are differences in perception between the social classes as to what sort of measures will make the child safe. Perhaps some groups of mothers think that bought equipment will be a more effective safeguard than one devised at home. Health education literature and shops like Mothercare promote bought equipment. Yet a heavy sofa is probably as good as a socket cover as a guard against electrical accidents. Gates cause hazards of their own since children try to climb over them and fall, or run against them in their play.

Some people may argue that not to buy a safety seat for the car or a fireguard indicates that parents are either ignorant of the risk or give safety care low priority. But on balance ownership of safety gadgets must surely be seen in the context of the mothers' interventionist approach to safety care and the urgency and force with which they discussed it. They took safety precautions but not necessarily the most expensive ones – and the poorer parents had other pressing claims on their income.

Road risks

As we noted earlier, accidental death to under-fives is mainly from road accidents, as pedestrians, hit by motorized traffic. And there is a strong relationship with occupational class. Mothers and children tend to be pedestrians rather than car riders (c.f. Graham, 1984). Few women have the use of a car during the day, yet they and the children make many journeys – to shops, clinics, doctors, parks, playgroups or to visit friends and relatives. Of the 135 mothers, only a quarter had the use of the car during the week, almost all of them in classes I and II. Sixteen per cent of the households, mainly from classes IIIb, IV and V, lived on estates where cars and people used the same access routes. And while 22 per cent of classes I and II households lived near roads classed (by us) as particularly dangerous, 50 per cent of the other households did so. Living near a dangerous road is likely to increase the chance of a road accident. One study found that 74 per cent of road accidents to under-fives took place within a quarter of a mile from their homes (Russan, 1977).

So though all the mothers and children were exposed to risks from traffic, the socially disadvantaged households were disadvantaged in this respect too. How did mothers care for their children's safety on the roads? They all thought roads were a serious hazard and they all supervised their children. Two-fifths of them, equally from all social classes, used some kind of restraint (reins or push-chair), and this was mainly for the under-twos. After that children wanted to walk and run and some refused to be restrained. Mothers accepted this development and relied on supervising them. Some valued letting the child explore in order to learn safe behaviour – as noted earlier, this was more common among classes I and II – and these mothers faced a particular problem in balancing their beliefs against the children's road safety:

> A major problem which is heavily on my mind is the road because part of letting him explore is – I let him walk up and down the road. He gets the idea where there's a pavement, but where there's no pavement – in a dip in the pavement, he rushes down to the road. He looks at me, he knows it's naughty but not that it's dangerous. He knows because sometimes I say stop or smack him and say that's very naughty, or sometimes I put him in the pushchair. But he wants to walk. Today coming home from the clinic he suddenly charged out towards the road. It's being naughty, rather than having a battle. He's not trying to fight me. He's not at that stage. He's not proving a point. I can always stop him. There's much more overseeing now though, just because he's mobile.

However, most of the mothers valued supervision above other methods of learning. They tried to hold onto their children, who sometimes broke free ('She tore away from us and ran ahead of us, straight out into the road'). The main problems were that their children were now highly mobile, adventurous, in some cases 'naughty' or 'defiant', and above all they did things so suddenly and so fast that parents could not always prevent dangerous behaviour in the street.

> It's a problem, crossing the road. He's very naughty – he won't hold your hand – he's very independent – we're having a battle with him at the moment. You have to lunge after him to grab him back.

Discussion

Mothers were keenly aware of safety problems and were interventionist in their approach to safety care. Much thought, worry and effort went in to safety care. There was no doubt that safety had high priority. The proviso to this is that a few mothers (10, or 7 per cent) seemed to us to overemphasize supervision at the expense of preventive care. There were no discernible class differences between mothers in their approaches to safety care nor in the strategies they adopted, either singly or in combination with others.

But it was only too clear that parents in poor housing were severely constrained in their ability to safeguard their children, because the housing had unalterable dangerous features. The interviews also suggested that poverty was a factor that constrained parents from buying safety gadgets.

Mothers in poor housing had to choose between health and safety. They restricted active exploratory play to safeguard their children. For some mothers child care involved endlessly rebuking and restraining their children within a dangerous environment. Then the children became defiant or the mother perceived them to be so. This situation contrasts with that of more affluent mothers living in a spacious child-proofed home, who were able to let their children behave much more as they chose. The data here highlight the relevance of considering people's behaviour in the light of their circumstances. Indeed it can be argued that to make a division between background circumstances and behaviour and to study their relative importance is to miss a central point – that people behave in certain ways not only because of beliefs, but because of a wide number of factors that feed into a complex process of decision-making. As regards safety care, some at least of these factors were characteristics of the housing, dangers in the neighbourhood, what safety devices were best given the household income, the child's level of activity and developmental stage, and how well she understood about dangers.

What interventions are appropriate to help reduce the toll of accidents to young children? Some commentators opt for health education for parents; for teaching them how to supervise and what gadgets are appropriate. No parents may find it helpful to be alerted to safety care problems and to be pointed towards ways of dealing with them. Some research suggests that children who have accidents are likely to have poor relationships with their parents (see Calnan and Wadsworth, 1977, for review). If so, then the evidence described here suggests environmental factors are relevant. But the weight of evidence provided by mothers in this study, as in others, supports the argument that intervention to improve housing and financial resources is needed to help parents keep their children safe (c.f. Townsend and Davidson, 1982; OHE, 1981; Blaxter, 1981).

Finally, some of the comments quoted in this chapter suggest the intimate knowledge mothers had of their child. This knowledge was important in other aspects of their health care of their children, as noted in other chapters (e.g. 6, 7 and 8). To conclude, here are some mothers talking about their children. They show the detailed, finely tuned understanding mothers had of their children: of their characters; of the type of knowledge they had; of their ability, or not, to generalize; of their memory; and of the extent to which they relied on their parents. It was through mothers' understanding of these factors, and of how each was changing daily that mothers chose to adopt and adapt various strategies of safety care.

> He's just starting to know when something's hot. If I've got a mug of coffee and I say it's hot – he won't touch it. But on the other hand, if he saw the mug without my being there and it was steaming, he might just touch it. He has no conception of it generally.

> I think she's got – it's really whether they've got a natural instinct as to what's dangerous. She's aware of all those things (hot taps, plugs, steam, stairs). She is cautious in those areas. And she'll tell *me* if I'm doing it wrong. She doesn't do any of those things – but of course you never risk it. You rely on the child's integrity, but you never rely on the child, because there's always that one occasion.

> He knows the iron's hot and the oven, he sometimes remembers not to stand in the bath except on the rubber mat. I think he understands he has to stay on that. I've told him, that's how he knows. He doesn't eat things, put things in his mouth as much as he did – that's just getting older. So he's safer in that respect. I still can't drum it into his head that he mustn't jump on the beds because he could fall off. It doesn't occur to him that it's dangerous.

> He's very cautious – he doesn't take any risks at all, so he must be aware of risks, or in a general way he's a bit of a coward. For example he never shuts his fingers in drawers or doors. But then he never did. He's not brave. He could fall downstairs or off the wall (in the

garden). That's because he's got no knowledge – he could take a step off because he doesn't know there's a gap. But on the stairs, if he's alone he's very cautious. If he's with you, holding your hand – he'll just step straight off.

Note to Chapter 4

1 On safety gadgets: there were significant differences by class for these: socket covers; cooker safeguards (guard or gate); fireguards (if there was a radiant fire); car seats (if the household had a car). There were significant differences by income for cooker safeguards; socket covers; and non-significant tendencies in the same direction for fireguards, gates and car seats.

5

Keeping Children Healthy

Introduction

This chapter is about mothers' perspectives on what constitutes good health in children, how to maintain it and how to prevent ill health. It shows that mothers had high standards in child health and saw health promotion and illness prevention as their responsibility, to be met within the resources of the household.

The chapter points to a wide range of actions and concerns that make up health care, and suggests that parental behaviours and concerns one might assume were directed to other ends are perceived by mothers as pertinent or crucial to the promotion of optimal health in their children. Thus, providing a loving secure home was seen not just as normal parental behaviour, but as a crucial determinant of good health. And food, similarly, was not given merely for survival and growth, but was perceived, if it was 'good' food, as a factor leading to the best of health in children. So keeping children in good health was work that was being consciously carried out when mothers engaged in many activities: giving them love and comfort, playing with and stimulating them, giving them rest and exercise, feeding them and keeping them clean. In this sense, then, the work of health promotion and maintenance was a central concern for mothers.

Mothers knew how to keep their children healthy and thought it was their job to do so. These perceptions provide a challenge to the commonly expressed view that some mothers lack knowledge and some also lack motivation to care well for their children. Such views are often supported by reference to some women's 'poor' preventive care practices for themselves, such as smoking.

What is Good Health?

Asked to describe a child in the very best of health, virtually all the mothers (except 5) gave a positive answer. That is, they saw good health as different from and better than an absence of illness. They talked about a child who looked clear-eyed, bright-faced, enthusiastic, active and investigative. It seemed that they expected of a healthy child that she should be reaching full potential – not just being without symptoms or disease, but raring to go, and, as mothers said, 'at it' and 'into everything'. There was also a suggestion that a child in the best of health would be developing, that is gaining in knowledge and physical ability and strength through exploration of the environment and through interaction with people around her. And a healthy child was one who ate well and slept well.

These descriptions echo what mothers said about specific aspects of health care. The data on safety care showed that mothers found it difficult to contain and safeguard their children, because of their active and exploratory behaviour. Yet mothers saw this behaviour as normal and desirable in itself, and those who lived in cramped housing said their children did not get enough exercise: 'She's all cramped up here; she can't run about. I have to take her out to the park every day'. And in a later chapter (8) it becomes clear that it was often changes in their children's appearance and levels of activity and in their appetite that led mothers to think the child was ill. Typically they would say the child became pale, or bleary-eyed, that she slowed down, or just flopped down, and often ate much less well than usual. The mothers' judgement was based on a comparison between signs of optimal health and deviations from it.

Here are some representative descriptions of a child in the best of health:

> Healthy child – lively, eating well, running around, chatting, some colour, clear-eyed, not tired-looking, a happy child. (*What do you think brings that about?*) Love from its parents, good food, exercise, playing in the open air, both parents keeping an eye on the child and noticing any changes in him; keeping the place clean and tidy.

Keeping Children Healthy

Healthy, well. Lively, jumping around (*What brings that about?*) Happiness. Being well looked after. Plenty of loving, that's the first thing. And plenty to eat.

Lively, alert, not over-weight or under-weight, bright eyes, not snivelly or grizzly. (*What brings that about?*) Apart from physical well-being, it's good food, caring for him, keeping him clean. People who care about him, give him attention, stimulate him.

A child who's alert and happy, bright-eyed, interested in what's going on around them. (*What brings that about?*) Stimulation. Talking to them, playing with them; being generally responsive to a child's needs and also being happy in yourself.

A healthy child — he's alert, getting into mischief. (*What brings that about?*) Proper meals, plenty of loving, and rest. That's it!

A generally healthy child — if he hasn't got a cold, and — he suffers from eczema — if he's not itching with it, and he hasn't got a cold, I'd say he was generally healthy. I get it you see — it's hereditary. It plays him up quite a bit. But if he's not itching I'd say he was healthy. If he was bright and alert and happy. You know if he's ill — if he cries you know there's a reason. If he's well he's happy. (*What brings that about?*) What they eat and how you look after them? What parents do, how you are with them, as long as you don't put too much pressure on them. It affects their moods then.

No illness, playful, not down, happy, eating well. (*What brings that about?*) Making sure he's washed, bathed, fed, has the right amount of sleep.

Nice complexion, not a sallow complexion, a clear complexion, not too fat. Active. Eats well. (*What brings that about?*) Good parents. Looking after them generally, not too fussy, make sure they have the right food, the essential vitamins, not giving too much bottle food as babies; I breast fed John. Good diet, good home background, bringing them up right, not letting them run wild, keeping an eye on them all the time.

It seemed that virtually all the mothers had high standards of good health for their children. Their descriptions did not sound like the equivalent for children of what some commentators have reported for adults: where a person defines herself as healthy if she can get through the day's tasks or duties, as Blaxter and Paterson (1982) found for some of their working class mothers in Aberdeen. Our mothers' vision of good health for their children approximates more nearly to the well-known definition adopted as an ideal by the WHO: 'Health is a state of complete physical, mental and social well-being, and not merely the absence of disease or infirmity'. If it is the case that people vary in their concepts of good health and that some have a low or negative standard: that is, they think of health as the absence of illness, or in terms mainly of their ability to get through the day, then we perhaps have to ask why was there such unanimity among our 135 mothers and such a positive concept of health for children. Do people in general think differently about what constitutes good health for a child, compared to their views on good health in adults? Is it that the range of things small children do is narrower than it is for adults and so we can agree more nearly with each other about what they should be doing? Do we also have a clearer idea about what a healthy child should look like, whereas we would find it difficult to describe a healthy adult? Is it also that most children have nothing wrong with them, whereas most adults have some sort of weakness, disability or long-term condition or feel that there might be a recurrence of some condition or that they are at risk of one that runs in the family or that tends to strike at a particular age or life-stage (c.f. Calnan and Johnson, 1985).

One way of looking at the problem is as follows. There is bound to be variation between people in their health but this variation is a matter of concern when it affects some groups (for instance, class groups). Ill health in childhood is of particular concern because it is class related and because of its possible long-term influences. As Blaxter (1981) notes, statistics are routinely kept on such things as average height and the range of normal development in children. So there are standards and measures for good health in children, whereas for adults we have no similar measures. From the child's birth onwards, mothers have before them a view of the child as having tasks to perform, not least because health visitors and doctors and leaflets at the clinic promote the view that there are weights to be achieved (for babies) and milestones to be reached. The child is supposed to be spending its time, initially gaining weight, then learning first to sit, then to crawl, to speak a word, then a sentence, to hold a cup, build a tower, climb the stairs and tie shoe-laces. Health professionals will define a child as healthy if she does well on the criteria they set out. So mothers have models of what a child's achievements should be and of how her days should be spent. These models feed into and help to mould their ideas of what a healthy child should be and should be doing. By contrast, there are probably few agreed or widely held models of how adults should spend their days and what goals they should strive towards.

Another point is that at the day-to-day level of health care described for us by mothers, it was clear that many of their views of what is normal, or worrying were derived from discussion with other mothers. Mothers build up a picture of what a healthy child is like by comparison with other children and what their mothers say about them (c.f. Buswell, 1983). People do not spend time doing this sort of comparative study on adults or not so intensively and not with such an urgent desire to know whether others or they themselves are healthy, according to local or national norms.

Keeping Children in Good Health

What brings about a state of positive health in a child? We thought initially that mothers' ideas on this would be of two kinds and that most mothers would probably hold both kinds. First, we thought people would refer to factors broadly out of their own control: such as luck, a naturally good constitution, or a good physical environment. Secondly, they would think their care of the child affected health status. In fact, mothers overwhelmingly emphasized the second of these two sorts of factors (see the examples on p. 76–7). Almost all (89 per cent) talked about the physical care of the child that parents give: nutrition, rest and exercise, hygiene and other preventive care actions. And most (73 per cent) thought psychological care of the child was crucial for the maintenance of good health; half (53 per cent) described the importance of providing a happy, loving and secure home and a third (34 per cent) said it was important to give the child interesting, stimulating and varied experiences. All but two of the 135 mothers talked in terms of physical or psychological care by parents, and the two most popular factors leading to good health were food (80 per cent) and a loving home (53 per cent). Smaller proportions referred as well to non-management factors – that is factors that in practical terms lay beyond their immediate control: fresh air (25 per cent), a good physical environment (12 per cent) or a naturally good or inherited constitution (11 per cent) (see Table 5.1).

Table 5.1 *Proportion of mothers who mentioned various factors contributing to optimal health in children*

Management
  Psychological care
    Loving home   53 ⎫
    Stimulation   34 ⎭ one or both – 73 ⎫
  (No. who gave this kind of answer only = 9)   ⎪
                                                        ⎬ both kinds
  Physical management   ⎪ of answer 64
    Food   80 ⎫
    Rest/exercise   32 ⎪ one or more – 89 ⎪
    Hygiene   16 ⎬
    Preventive care   13 ⎭
  (No. who gave this kind of answer only – 27)

Non-management
  Fresh air   25
  Good physical environ-
    ment   12
  Natural health   11
  (No. who gave this kind of answer only = 2)

No. of mothers = 135.

Mothers did not differ by class in what, broadly, they thought promoted optimal health: psychological care, good physical management or factors outside their control. But among management factors there were class differences. Many fewer mothers in classes IV and V compared to other mothers favoured food, and there was an increase in the numbers of mothers who favoured hygiene, between class I and classes IV and V.

It seemed therefore that virtually all the mothers saw the promotion of their children's good health as dependent on the care parents give them. And the kinds of care they thought important were essentially lay kinds of care. That is they were things ordinary people could do, and they were not actions either directly or indirectly influenced by health professionals. In other words, the mothers' views were not medicalized. None of them thought optimal health came about from the child being 'under the doctor' and none suggested that vitamins or tonics would bring about optimal health. As this study shows, mothers thought the care of their children lay in their hands, and they called in professional help when and if they saw fit. Doctors could offer advice and prescriptions for ill children, but the care of an ill child and the promotion of good health both rested with parents.

Clearly the mothers wanted to keep their children healthy and it seems fair to say that they were virtually all thinking in terms of health promotion as well as illness prevention. It is difficult to draw a conceptual distinction between the two, but health promotion can perhaps best be seen as concerned with the maintenance or enhancement of an existing state of health, in contrast to preventive activities where the emphasis is on the avoidance of ill health. The idea of health promotion is useful here in focusing attention on an aspect of parental child care which may mark it out from the characteristics of most adults' self-care.

Distinctions between promotion and prevention are in some ways easier to see in the case of parental care of young children than in the case of self-care by adults. Most children can be seen as starting off healthy, so maintenance of that position is more obviously appropriate than in the case of adults where experience of illness may lead people to concentrate on preventing the recurrence of illness or the deterioration of the present position. Then children grow (unlike adults!) and their bodies can be seen as needing food and exercise for that growth. The quality of the food and exercise can be seen as important to ensure extra good growth, giving them a good start. It is more difficult to see why food and exercise may promote health in full grown people. Thirdly, some of these mothers saw a close link between children's emotional security and their health. For half the mothers a child could be deemed healthy only if she was secure and happy in the love given by her parents. The link-up of ideas seems to be that a healthy child is one who functions well and this means being lively, among other things; liveliness in children depends at least partly on emotional health. Of course many people, including many of these mothers, think that adults can fall ill because of stress or depression, but people's definitions of a healthy adult probably vary widely, and the links between emotional well-being and health are less widely agreed.

Many of the practices mothers thought important for their children's health seemed promotional. For instance, giving children fresh air or a run in the park or good food or regular rest were seen as child-care practices with a dual promotional purpose: these actions enhanced the present good state of health; and they gave the child the opportunity to build up health for the future. Mothers talked about how much better the child was for outdoor exercise and fresh air (especially country air), and their emphasis was on the child's improved liveliness, temper and life-style – she ate and slept the better for it. Fresh air and exercise would lead to stronger limbs and a more active mind. A secure home with loving parents would allow a child the confidence to investigate the world – which was what a healthy child did.

Preventing Bad Health

How to prevent ill health seems a more difficult topic than how to promote good health. You can see a child's glowing face when you have given her a run in the park, but keeping a child warm to prevent illness merely maintains the status quo – and is not always successful. Promotion enhances and prevention maintains the child's health status. Mothers' descriptions of health care provided a variety of clues to their ideas on the causation and prevention of illness.

Causes of illness

Mothers described their children's recent illnesses (see Chapter 8 for more detail). Their accounts showed that they thought in terms of two principal kinds of cause for illness: first, infections of various kinds: germs, viruses, contagion, infection; and second, the effects of temperature change or of extremes of temperature – a spell of hot or cold weather, or the child being suddenly exposed to temperature change – through draughts, going out into the cold and so on. Fifty-nine per cent of mothers drew on germ theory and 35 per cent on thermal theories to account for one or more of their children's recent illnesses. Mothers in classes I and II were very much more likely than others to opt for germ theory. About a third of mothers in each class opted for thermal theories, except in classes IV and V where 58 per cent did so.

Causation and prevention of colds

Another kind of information on causation of illness was provided by answers to direct questions. We asked all mothers how they thought you caught a cold and whether they did anything to prevent colds — for their children or for themselves. Their comments suggest again that there were competing ideas in circulation among mothers. They used germ theory and thermal theory to explain how you catch a cold, and some mothers used both theories. Giving good food and keeping the child warm were the main ways of preventing colds; again some mothers held that both were useful.

Cause: You catch colds from other people — it's viruses.
Prevention: Give him a proper diet, and enough sleep. Try to keep him away from people who obviously have colds.

Cause: It's a germ, a virus. I don't believe it's through being cold.
Prevention: I wrap up warm against a cold. But colds don't come from getting cold — I keep telling my Mum — she's convinced they do. She says you'll catch cold from not keeping your cardigan on. He's got a little bit of a cold now. It started over a week ago. We went to our caravan on the East coast. It's very windy down there. Being down there in the cold probably brought it on. He got so sweaty running about and he wouldn't even have a cardigan on and it's so cold down there. I gave him vitamin drops against colds up to the end of this winter, but not now he's older.

Cause: Just normal contact and bugs in the area.
Prevention: Not for me. For her, just the normal precautions of wrapping her up when we go out. I put on what I think's right for me and then I ask her if she's cold and she just — you can't tell if she's hot or cold, so I just dress her up to be warm.

Cause: Various things. I wash my hair and catch a cold if I go out. Or she might pick it up from another child. She might run outside with nothing on and catch a cold.
Prevention: I give her fresh orange. And haliborange tablets, and malt extract — cod liver oil — when we remember.

Cause: It's things going through the air, off other people.
Prevention: No. I don't do anything. I can't remember her ever having a cold I remember she had a runny nose once.

Cause: It's from the changeable weather we have in the country. You have a fairly good day with the sun out and then it's cold in the evening. You get it because the change is too sudden for you.
Prevention: I never leave the windows open at night if it's breezy and I never let him out with light clothes on if it's a breezy day. I never have a cold house.

Cause: It's a virus I think.
Prevention: I make sure he doesn't get damp. And diet, give them the right kind of food. Otherwise they don't have enough resistance.

Cause: It's a bad virus. You can't help getting it if it's going round.
Prevention: No. You can't.

I never understood why he got all those colds in his first year. So I put it down to visitors bringing germs. But he never went round with nothing on, or was subject to draughts. He had proper care and good food.

Cause: From other children. If you don't dress your children up warm enough they can get a chill.
Prevention: I give him his children's vitamins and make sure he's well dressed for any kind of weather.

Most mothers (79 per cent) thought that at least one factor leading to colds was infection – germs, viruses, contact with people who had colds. But 36 per cent thought that getting cold, or changes in body temperature were at least partly responsible and 16 per cent thought that both infections and temperature were relevant factors. Mothers in classes I, II and IIIa were very much more likely to mention germs as a cause of colds, compared to other mothers, and mothers in classes IIIb, IV and V were very much more likely than others to mention temperature change as a cause. Those who thought temperature was a causative factor tended to take steps to keep their children warm. Thirty-four per cent of mothers said they did this, equally by class. Most of those who thought infections were solely responsible for colds, said they did nothing to try to prevent them, because there was nothing that was likely to be effective (72 per cent of 54).

However, irrespective of what was thought to be the cause of colds, a proportion of the mothers (37 per cent) favoured giving children good food to prevent colds, especially food with vitamins in it or vitamins on their own. There was a very clear class difference on this, with a broad divide between classes I and II (60 per cent) and classes III, IV and V (21 per cent). So routine dietary supplements – which were not mentioned for promoting health – did feature as a means of preventing colds. The principal supplement was vitamin pills or drops; 24 per cent of mothers gave these to their children. Only two mothers gave, or tried to give, tonics (Minadex, Lucozade). In general, though, vitamins, especially vitamin C, whether in fruit, vegetables or as supplements, were the main dietary defence against colds.

Protecting the teeth

Keeping children's teeth in good condition was something all the mothers said they aimed for (see Chapter 7). What they said about how to protect teeth suggested ideas that are similar to those being considered here. There were two main ways of protecting teeth. The first was to clean them of dangerous substances, such as sticky and sweet food, or to avoid such foods in the first place. The second was to strengthen the teeth by giving the child calcium and fluoride. Everyone favoured the first of these procedures (cleaning the teeth) and 55 per cent favoured the second (building up the teeth). There was a class divide, with most mothers in classes I and II (66 per cent) favouring building while fewer other mothers (47 per cent) did so.

Promotion of Health and Prevention of Illness for Children

This survey across mothers' views on promoting health and preventing ill health in their children, suggests that for all mothers the key to good health lay in their care of their children, in the love and security they gave and in good management. Keeping children healthy meant giving good food, enough sleep and exercise, keeping them clean and warm. For few mothers did it mean using tonics or pills and then only to prevent illness rather than to promote health. So the health care of young children was a matter of commonsense and tradition. Resources within the home were what counted.

It also seems that there were two main kinds of explanation being proposed about why children stay well and get ill. On the first view the important thing was to build the child's strength and resistance, and this included strengthening the teeth. Food was particularly important for this and particular constituents of food – vitamins for preventing colds and calcium and fluoride for strengthening teeth. This view was held more strongly among mothers in classes I and II. They were also more likely to stress germ theory than other mothers, so possibly they thought the best way to prevent germs from affecting the child was by making the child strong.

On the second view, the emphasis was on protecting the child from what might come to the attack, not so much by building up the child's defences, as by warding off attack. Thus teeth were prevented from decay by cleaning off sweet and sticky foods. Children were protected from the cold weather, which could cause a cold, by wrapping them up warmly, and especially by keeping their heads warm. Good health was promoted and bad health deflected by good hygiene, which killed germs before they could attack. These more traditional views about causation and prevention of illness were more common in classes III, IV and V – and especially in IIIb, IV and V. This may be because these mothers, with less formal education, had knowledge handed down to them rather than book knowledge or knowledge put about by professionals.

Food was of central importance for promoting optimal health and for preventing ill health, including colds. Every mother (except 2) referred to food in connection with one or more of these promotive or preventive measures. Of the sorts of physical care mothers mentioned for promoting health, it was far and away the most popular.

It is interesting, however, that some groups of mothers stressed food more than others. There was a steady drop in number of mentions of food in connection with promotion and prevention, from class I to classes IV and V. This trend could reflect class differences in behaviour during an interview. For instance, middle-class mothers may think it appropriate to repeat and stress their views; working-class mothers may be less keen to promote their views; or be more succinct. But possibly the idea of food as central to health was particularly important among some class groups. Mothers' ideas about feeding their children, and their practices are considered in more detail in the next chapter.

Preventive Care – for Self and Child

The study focused on mothers' care of their children, not of themselves. But it threw light on an interesting contrast between self-care and child care. Almost all the mothers (87 per cent) said they took some action to prevent their children getting colds or illnesses in general. However a fifth of them (22 per cent) said they did not bother for themselves. They took preventive action for the child because she was more vulnerable, or because they cared more or worried more about her than they did about themselves. There was a fairly striking contrast between classes IIIb, IV and V and other mothers on this. Only half of them said they took some preventive action for themselves, compared to three-quarters of mothers in classes I, II and IIIa (48 per cent as against 76 per cent).

This finding is interesting because it feeds into the debate on whether there are class differences in perspectives on the value of preventive health actions. Some people argue that working-class people put low value on preventive health care for themselves and their children. Others that they lack access to knowledge of what practices are good for health. Various points can be made in the light of this study's findings.

The first point relates to the weight that can be put on the findings; possibly the class difference reflects only, or mainly, class differences in behaviour during an interview. Some mothers in classes IIIb, IV and V, more than other mothers, may have felt it appropriate to stress their care of their children to a middle-class interviewer, even to the extent of suggesting that they sacrificed themselves. So perhaps some down-played self-care. Other mothers may have been more aware that self-care is considered desirable – by the DHSS, the HEC and the media – and have talked to us with that in mind.

But, secondly, it seems probable that there was a group of mothers, defined broadly within class, who did feel preventive care for themselves was unimportant, at least compared to preventive child care. Probably some mothers do think they should do more for their children than for themselves, and that if it comes to a choice they will neglect themselves to care for their children. Such mothers were vividly described by Spring-Rice (1939) in her accounts of working class housewives and mothers, who gave themselves poor food and had chronic untreated conditions. Recently Graham (1985) has pointed to similar self-sacrifice among mothers living in poverty. While poorer mothers in our sample did refer to such choices, well-to-do mothers did not have to face them.

However, the data presented in this chapter suggest that all mothers were keen to promote good child health. So if mothers talked light-heartedly, off-handedly or self-sacrificially about preventive care for themselves, this cannot be taken as indicative of their attitudes towards preventive care for their children. Yet this extrapolation is often made. Studies of mothers' preventive care practices have found that those who, for instance, smoke or do not have smear tests are also those who do not take their children to the clinic for preventive services. The inference has been made that the mother devalues preventive care for both self and child. This inference is made on the assumption that mothers give the same value to self-care as to child care; but, as suggested here, the assumption may be unfounded. The inference also assumes that reasons for 'poor' practices are the same for self-care as for child care. But the reasons may differ. Women may neglect themselves because they are busy, unhappy or devalue their own health; whereas they may stop going to the child health clinic because they know their child is well and they have no need for a professional opinion, or because the clinic service is perceived as poor.

Mothers' Health Care Work – Implications for Professionals

This chapter has pointed to some of the many health care actions mothers perceive as important determinants of their children's health status. Some characteristics of their perspectives have implications for the work of those to whom parents turn for help. First, many of their actions derive from their unique knowledge of what works for that child, that is from knowledge gained from continuous committed care of the child. Secondly, these health care actions are perceived essentially as ones that parents carry out within the resources of the household and which form part of the normal patterns of behaviour within that household. These points suggest that professionals do well to recognize and respect mothers' perspectives. Their help is likely to be acceptable and useful only if they work within the assumption that mothers know what they are about and have worked out good ways of caring for their children.

Mothers also indicated that, like everyone, they carry round with them a mixed bag of knowledge, probably derived from various sources: some bits learned in childhood, some tacked on after watching television or talking to the doctor, others learned from experience. It was particularly striking that on the causation and prevention of colds some people argued on two or more fronts. It is often suggested that when health professionals meet people, a professional, or medical set of explanations meet a lay set. Whether professional people, such as doctors, actually do have a perfectly coherent set of professional beliefs unsullied by residual lay beliefs is open to question. Nevertheless the meeting may, and probably does, involve a negotiation within which the professional and the lay person seek agreement on causation, processes and treatment. It is essential for professionals to be aware of the framework in which individual people operate and to work within that. Otherwise, again, their explanations and suggestions for action may well be unacceptable.

Finally, this chapter on concepts of health care may help readers to understand mothers' health care in specific areas and the choices they make. It may contribute to understanding of the *conflicts* mothers face in their health care work, and how they have to choose between *priorities*. It was noted in Chapter 4 that two aims in health care may conflict: the aim of keeping children safe and the aim of facilitating healthy activity and exploration. Once one understands that activity and exploration are seen as health promoting, then it becomes easier to understand why some accidents take place and what is *not* an appropriate professional response. Thus one mother told how she and her husband watched their child climbing on the mantel-piece (exploration) and stood ready to catch him if he fell. He fell and cut his head. The nurse and doctor at the hospital kept saying, but why did you let him climb? For the parents, these comments were inappropriate and hurtful: they had made positive health choices; perhaps, with hindsight, not the best, but positive choices. How mothers feed their children and care for their teeth are also health work topics which can best be understood in the context of ideas about health promotion and maintenance. Again mothers have to make choices between various conflicting aims and in response to various pressures. The next two chapters explore these two topics.

6

Feeding the Children

Introduction

In Chapter 5 it was shown that promoting children's health is a central focus of mothers' work. A major factor contributing to good health was food; indeed every mother thought food relevant for health maintenance or illness prevention. Many mothers also stressed that good health consisted of both physical and emotional well-being. This chapter shows how mothers took both these kinds of well-being into account when feeding their children.

The chapter starts by describing children's diets and considers similarities and differences between groups of children, according to both age and class. It goes on to consider what factors affected what the children ate. Mothers' food choices take place in the context of a wide range of considerations and pressures. They choose 'good' food, that is, food that promotes physical health, and food that is good because it is established and accepted in the household. What they can afford determines food choice; so does what is available locally, what is advertised and what is promoted in the shops. They decide on certain foods and meals in the context of what the day's events and crises suggest; they take into account their own and their children's social life. Children themselves establish their own preferences and routines, and some of their daily food is given by other caregivers. So already these young children's diets are affected by many factors beyond the control of individual mothers.

Consideration of mothers' accounts of how they feed their children suggests that their criteria for good food may be less influential in determining their children's diets than a variety of other pressures. Notably, people's access to good food may matter more than their perceptions of good food. This is obviously an important topic, because diet affects health. Currently, certain popular foods such as fats and sugars are identified by nutritionists as leading to obesity which in turn is thought to be associated with a long list of health problems – heart conditions, liver and kidney disease and varicose veins. Sugar is widely thought to promote dental decay. So it is important to consider what kinds of intervention are likely to improve children's diets; broadly, intervention to educate mothers, or intervention to facilitate people's access to certain types of food. This is the policy context within which the mothers' accounts are considered.

What the Children Ate 'Yesterday'

Mothers told us what their children ate all day 'yesterday' from first thing in the morning to last thing at night. This provided a list of occasions when food or drinks was consumed and a list of items consumed.[1] 'Yesterday' was in almost every case a weekday (because we avoided interviews on Sundays and Mondays) so the data are about everyday routines and patterns, not about weekends. Even so, 'yesterday' was varied in character: a few children had birthdays, or went to parties; some were ill, or being difficult; there were visitors, expeditions and crises. In four cases the mother knew little about the day's food because the child was with someone else for most of the day. But the picture we have for 131 children allows us to see different patterns of food intake and to consider relationships between these patterns and factors that may have affected them.

The mothers talked freely and with a good deal of 'colour' about feeding their children. Their accounts have both advantages and disadvantages. They are probably fairly complete, but do not allow for analysis of quantity. We settled for recording the number of portions of types of food children had, and made out for ourselves a guide for deciding which foods were sugared or high in fat.

Table 6.1 shows the day's food intake for 131 children. Some foods were more popular than others. Most of the children had cereals several times a day and potatoes or other root vegetables

Table 6.1 *General picture: proportion of children who consumed types of food 'yesterday' (%)*

	\multicolumn{8}{c}{Number of portions/occasions}
	0	1	2	3	4	5	6	7+
Cereals (bread, rice, cornflakes, pastry)	1	5	15	25	28	12	8	8
Starchy fruit & vegetables (bananas, turnips, carrots, potatoes, rice, crisps, chips)	17	39	32	7	5	0	1	0
Legumes (peas, beans)	57	37	5	1	0	0	0	0
Cooked leafy vegetables (cabbage, cauliflower, sprouts, 'greens', spinach)	80	18	2	1	0	0	0	0
Fresh, uncooked fruit & vegetables (tomatoes, lettuce) (including unsweetened fruit juice)	41	18	15	6	6	2	2	9
Cooked fruit (tinned, in puddings, jam)	64	29	6	1	0	0	0	0
Eggs	61	34	5	1	0	0	0	0
Meat	17	53	23	6	1	0	0	0
Fish	82	17	1	0	0	0	0	0
Milk alone (including milk drinks, hot chocolate)	16	28	27	18	3	3	1	5
Milk in cereals/drinks	19	42	22	10	3	1	4	0
Other milk produce (butter, cheese, yoghurt)	12	28	35	19	5	2	0	0
Sweets, chocolate/icecream	58	31	8	3	1	0	0	0
Cakes/biscuits	41	33	18	3	4	1	0	0
Crisps, chips	59	28	11	2	1	0	0	0
Sweet drinks (orange squash, fizzy drinks, tea/coffee with sugar)	27	15	11	13	7	6	1	21

All rows sum to 100%. Number of children = 131.

or a banana. If cereals and starchy food and legumes are put together, as 'starchy foods', then 15 per cent of the children had 1, 2 or 3 portions, 51 per cent 4, 5 or 6 portions and 37 per cent seven or more. Fish and cooked green vegetables were the least popular foods. Fish, except for fish fingers, seems not to have figured in mothers' shopping baskets. However, almost every child (except 9 who were ill) had meat, fish or eggs 'yesterday' (32 per cent one portion, 37 per cent two, 24 per cent three or more). No child was being brought up as a vegetarian, though some mothers were themselves vegetarian. Cooked green vegetables were unpopular with the children and many mothers said they had ceased to offer them to their child. Many children had no fresh fruit or vegetables, and what they did have was often in the form of cartoned or frozen fruit juice. If fresh (raw) fruit, including juice, and vegetables and cooked green vegetables are put together, then 32 per cent had none, 24 per cent one portion/drink, 16 per cent two and 28 per cent more. A high proportion had no milk on its own or just one drink of milk (44 per cent), but every child except two had milk in some form, though it might just be in cups of tea. Most of the children had sugar many times a day and most had several foods high in cholesterol. Adding these two sorts of food together gave a score of foods that are thought to be fattening. (Foods high in both sugar and cholesterol were counted twice.) Eight per cent of children scored less than 5, 43 per cent scored 5–9, 22 per cent scored 10–14, and 27 per cent had 15 or more items of food high in sugar and/or cholesterol.

Sugar was an important part of the diet for most children. Three-quarters of them had some sort of sweetened drink – tea, coffee, squash or canned or bottled fizzy drinks, and 94 per cent had sweetened food of some kind. If all sweetened drinks and sweetened items of food are put together then 5 per cent had none, 13 per cent had one, 26 per cent two or three, 28 per cent 4, 5 or 6 and 38 per cent seven or more.

A fifth of the children (21 per cent) had squash-type drinks on demand all day, or a bottle or mug of squash topped up all day long. It is interesting that sweets, chocolate and icecream do not account for much of the sweetened food. Only 12 per cent of the children had them twice or more. Similarly a quarter of the children had cake or biscuits twice or more. But sugar comes in many other foods, for instance in jam, in yoghurt, and on cereals and all these were popular with the children.

Sweetened drinks seem to occupy a privileged position in some mothers' minds. People who said they tried to avoid giving sugar would talk cheerfully about orange squash. Perhaps, as the advertisers would wish, people think it is good because of the vitamins, rather than bad because of the sugar. One mother said, 'I try not to give him too many sweet things, because of his teeth' but then she explained that the child had drinks on demand:

he has a cup and we just keep filling it up all day with whatever he wants. He'll go into the kitchen and point to what he wants. There's milk, Ribena, strawberry cordial, lemonade, orange squash, tea, coffee.

A high proportion of children (28 per cent) had seven or more sugared meals/snacks, including 21 per cent who had literally a countless number – because they had sweetened drinks on the go all day. Most mothers (69 per cent) said they tried to restrict sugar, but they noted how difficult that was. Some of the problems are discussed later.

There was a wide variation in the number of occasions on which children had food and/or drink. Here is one child's food intake for the day:

		Varieties of food
First thing	cup of tea and milk	2
Breakfast	Weetabix and milk and sugar; tea	2
Went out	sweets on the way to Nan's	1
At Nan's, mid-day	piece of ham, bread and butter; tea	3
At playgroup	orange squash and biscuit	2
On the way home	iced lolly	1
5.30 p.m. dinner	steak and kidney pie, potato, peas, cake, tea	7
6.45 p.m.	piece of an orange; biscuit	1
7.30 p.m.	chocolate given by grandfather	1
8.30 p.m. in bed	bottle of milk	1
		21

plus cups of tea (with milk, no sugar) all day, whenever adults had one. (Note that each variety of food is counted at its first appearance; milk on its own is counted separately from milk in drinks/with cereals.)

This little girl, aged nearly three, had her main meal in the evening. Her mother said she usually just gave her a snack midday, and various cakes and biscuits and crisps through the day; her grandparents gave her sweets and chocolate too. She had food or drink ten times 'yesterday', plus uncountable cups of tea. ('Uncountable' means that the mother could not count them, but she said they were more than six.) She had 21 varieties of food, and eight sugared items; seven of her meals/snacks had sugar in them.

Another, younger child (aged 21 months) had her main meal in the middle of the day. She had six meals/snacks, of which four had sweet food in them. She had 17 varieties of food.

		Varieties of food
8 a.m.	orange juice, bit of apple	
	Ready-Brek and milk and honey	5
At the shops	piece of cheese and some nuts	2
1.30 p.m.	mincemeat with carrots, mashed	
	potato, icecream, milk	5
Mid-afternoon	orange juice; half a fruit bun	1
6 p.m.	bread and peanut butter; fruit yoghurt	4
7-ish	milk	
		17

These two children had many different kinds of food 'yesterday'; they had protein, carbohydrate and vitamins, or to put it another way they had meat, milk, cereals and fruit. They probably both got enough of the kinds of foods professionals recommend for children's health. One child had her meal at mid-day, the other in the evening – and they ate and drank on several other occasions.

A third child (aged 22 months) had a more limited menu 'yesterday':

		Varieties of food
Breakfast	tea and milk (would not eat cereal)	2
11.45 a.m.	sausage roll, baked beans, milk	4
5 p.m. dinner	boiled potato, mincemeat, fizzy ginger	
	drink	3
9 p.m.	toasted cheese, milk, tea and milk	2
		11

This child had food on only four occasions, and she had few varieties of food, with no fruit or green vegetables. Her mother said she liked to give her daughter main meals rather than snacks, because they were better for her, and that the child ate the same food as they did.

These examples show something of the variety of children's diets, and of the distribution of food through the day. The mothers thought in terms of main meals, other meals, or light meals, and snacks, and they reckoned to give their children a main meal each day.

Table 6.2 *Varieties of food and meals/snacks consumed 'yesterday'*

	Varieties of food							
	7,8	9,10	11,12	13,14	15,16	17,18	19,20	21–33
% of children	5	13	15	21	19	15	7	5

	Number of meals and snacks								
	3	4	5	6	7	8	9	10	11	countless
% of children	2	4	18	21	12	5	8	1	3	25

Rows sum to 100%. Number of children = 131.

Table 6.2 shows the wide range in numbers of foods, and numbers of occasions when food was eaten. A third of the children had up to 12 varieties and 27 per cent had 17 or more. A quarter had food no more than five times in the day, while 37 per cent had food nine times or more, including the children who had countless drinks during the day. Overall, it is clear that providing food is a major activity in a mother's day.

Class Differences in Children's Diet 'Yesterday'

There were clear differences here. Moving along the class continuum from I to IV and V, children had very many fewer portions of fresh fruit and vegetables, more crisps and chips, more foods that were both sugared and high in cholesterol. And they had more sugared meals and snacks through the day. But there were no differences between children from different class households as to how many protein, starchy or carbohydrate foods or varieties of food they had. This picture bears out a prevalent view that children get enough of the various kinds of food they need for health (though the quality of the protein may vary), except for fruit and vegetables. In addition some get a lot of sugary and fatty foods.

Within class groups there were interesting contrasts according to the child's age. Children in classes I, II and IIIa, whatever their age, had much the same amount of milk, fruit and vegetables, and sugared and fatty foods. But in classes IIIb, IV and V there was a general tendency for the younger children to have better food than the older ones. Thus the older children in class IIIb had less fruit and vegetables and much less milk and older children in classes IV and V had more sugared food. It looks as if children in classes I, II and IIIa went on having much the same diets over the eighteen month age-range, but in classes IIIb, IV and V their diets changed as they got older.

To say there are such class differences, however, does not explain them. Many factors could be responsible for differences in children's diets, and there is unlikely to be any simple answer to the problem. Many factors will interact to produce a certain result. Mothers in classes I and II and to some extent also in class IIIa had high educational levels, compared to other mothers. But they also had higher incomes, probably more opportunity to choose certain foods, and probably sets of beliefs associated with patterns of behaviour within class groups. Any or all of these may have been important in affecting their children's diets, and these factors are examined here.

Income

Mothers said that their low income affected the children's diet. And analysis of data, setting the diets against household income, confirmed the picture. Eight mothers said that money problems affected what food they were able to give their children. In particular providing fruit and meat was sometimes beyond their means. Probably this was the tip of the iceberg. Mothers tend to feel guilty if they cannot feed their children as they would like and may not mention financial constraints. Some of the issues were explained by this mother:

> If you have bills to pay they have to come first. You have to have electricity, you have to pay the rent. I'd like to give her a variety of foods, rather than buying cheaper cuts. I'd prefer her to have fresh orange, not squash. Being luxurious with food – last year when my husband was in a better job I did do that. Fresh fruit every day, giving her the opportunity to try different foods – not having to worry about waste. She always has some sort of meat, every day, including chicken once a week. I'd like to give her beef but I can't always afford it.

Of the 135 households, 29 per cent had a net weekly income of less than £100, including 6 per cent on less than £65. So though many households were poor, few were at the extremes of poverty. Nevertheless, analysis of the diets of children in the poorer households (29 per cent of all) compared to the rest showed important differences. The children had fewer varieties of food than other children: only 18 per cent had 17 or more kinds of food, compared to 31 per cent of the rest. So they had less chance of getting all the constituents of food they needed. They filled up with biscuits and crisps more than other children. They had milk and milk products rather less often in the day. Most striking of all, they had very many fewer portions of fresh fruit and vegetables than other children. Fifty-three per cent had none and 29 per cent only one portion, compared to 23 per cent and 22 per cent for the others.

It seems obvious that low income will affect food choice and many surveys show differences in diet according to income (e.g. Food Policy Unit, 1984; Burnett, 1979; Burghes, 1980). But some people will argue that even on a low income mothers can provide good food if they know what is good and are strongly motivated. So it is important to consider other factors that affected food choice and to suggest ways in which low income was important in steering mothers towards giving certain sorts of food.

Food Choice – Health and Custom

We asked mothers *how they chose food for the children*. We did not direct the answers, beyond interpolating an occasional 'Why?', and mothers could and did give any sort of answer from a technical account of food values to 'it's what we have'. But something that may have affected mothers' replies was that the interview was mainly about promoting health and preventing illness. Almost all the mothers (91 per cent) said something health-related about their choice of food. They mentioned body-building, or protein (58 per cent), or they specifically referred to bone-building, or calcium (30 per cent); or they said they chose food because it had vitamins, which were good for health (59 per cent). A few mothers talked about carbohydrates, or energy-giving foods (19 per cent). Some mothers covered the field more generally with the word 'variety' or 'balance'; a varied or balanced diet would be likely to contain everything a child needed for her health (35 per cent). Some mothers thought fresh or natural food was healthy (32 per cent). Twenty-five per cent mentioned choosing foods that the child could digest easily, or which acted as roughage. And 9 per cent talked in more general terms about the protective or satisfying qualities of food – they thought food should be warming or filling.

There was a class difference between mothers on the type of health reasons they gave for food choice. Mothers in classes I, II and IIIa were more likely than others to mention protein, and carbohydrates or functions of these. This may be because they thought it appropriate to talk like this in an interview on health; it may be that more of them did have this kind of knowledge. There was no class difference on vitamins. They are probably the best known health 'ingredient' of food – advertisements for breakfast cereals boast of them; women are often urged to take them, for instance in pregnancy, and to give them to their young children. Overall, mothers in the manual workers' households gave fewer health reasons and gave more general ones – they referred to variety or balance.

A mother's choice of food for her household is likely to depend partly on the repertoire she brings to the job – the foods and meals she grew up with and sees as being normal and acceptable. In addition, the mother as main food provider takes into account the father's and children's preferences. Most of the mothers (68 per cent) talked in these terms about their approaches to food choice. For instance:

> I just usually choose what I used to have at home, what my mother cooked. I also cook what I like or what my husband likes. And I like trying out new recipes. I like cooking. Ninety-nine per cent of what the food is, is what I used to eat as a child. The rest is because I like cooking.

These mothers were emphasizing *family custom* and the value of food that is tried and tested. It has nourished children and adults in the past and thus proved its worth. Its nutritional content could be assumed. In addition, they were emphasizing the value of keeping up family traditions and the pleasure they took in providing and eating familiar meals. There was a class contrast here. Many more mothers in classes III, IV and V (79 per cent) talked in these terms, compared to those in classes I and II (53 per cent). And 14 per cent of class III, IV and V mothers talked *only* in terms of family custom, that is, they did not describe food choice at all in terms of its health-related importance, whether specifically or generally.

So mothers described the provision of food in terms of health and/or family custom and there was a broad division between the two main class groups on this. Of course this division is artificial in a way; it is partly a product of what we thought interesting in the data. On the other hand, it does account for some differences in diets. Some of the mothers (32 per cent) talked *only* in health terms about their choice of food (47 per cent in classes I and II and 21 per cent in classes III, IV and V) and children in these households had fewer sugared meals and snacks in the day compared to other children. This was independent of class. So it seems that mothers did carry through their spoken emphasis on health reasons into practice.

Catering for Children

The children (all aged 18–36 months) almost all had a diet similar to that of their parents, though some also had extra milk and baby foods. Regarding diet, the mothers were treating them as children rather than as babies. They took their child's views into account: over half the mothers (56 per cent) said they chose food at least partly because the child liked it, and 'yesterday' 55 per cent of the children had a specific meal or food because their mothers knew they liked it. By this age they had clear likes and dislikes, though, as mothers noted, these changed, often suddenly. Children's wishes were also met as regards snacks; they were given food when they asked for it, as a matter of routine or to keep them going, and this pattern was more firmly established among the older children.

Children were also allowed to choose whether or not to eat. 'Yesterday', 37 per cent of the children were said to have rejected something they were offered – a particular food or a whole meal. Most of their mothers (84 per cent) accepted this; either they offered the child something else or tried to make up for the rejected food, if they thought it was important, later in the day. There appears to have been a change since the 1960s when nearly half the mothers in a Nottingham study thought children should be pressured to eat what they were given (Newson and Newson, 1970, ch. 8, pp. 216–56).

There were no class differences on any of this. But there was a difference in ideas about meal-times which suggests that while most class III, IV and V mothers thought of meal-times as important occasions for father, mother and children to be together, many of the other mothers did not.

Meals

An important consideration in the choice of food and the provision of food for children through the day is what constitutes a good meal. It is a commonplace idea that people consider a good main meal consists of meat and two vegetables, and with some variations this was what most of the mothers (89 per cent) thought. A main meal for a child had protein (meat, fish or egg) and at least two vegetables (usually including potatoes, green vegetables, root vegetables or salad). A main meal was important for giving some of the important types of food and ingredients of food that children need; proteins or body-building foods, vitamins to protect them and filling food.

For 43 per cent of the mothers the best way to feed children was to concentrate their food into main meals, so as to be sure they got good food. Snacks were relatively worthless for health and, worse, they deterred the child from eating a main meal. However, 50 per cent of the mothers placed less reliance on the idea of a main meal, and argued instead for making sure the child got what she needed, whether that was in snacks or in main meals. Some of these mothers were arguing from their knowledge of their child, who was happier eating smaller amounts at shorter intervals, or did not like the sort of food provided for a main meal. And a small proportion (7 per cent) argued that for their child snacks were *better* than meals because the child so much preferred them.

What mothers said about the value of main meals versus snacks depended on their child's age. Fifty-eight per cent of mothers with an under-two favoured main meals compared to 32 per cent of those with an over-two. It seemed that mothers started off aiming for main meals but changed their minds or their practices as the child developed a taste for snacks and made her own wishes known.

There were no differences between class groups on any of this. There was, however, a clear class divide in mothers' ideas about *when* the child should have main meals, and these ideas affected the child's diet as a whole. For most mothers in classes I and II (59 per cent), the child's main meal was at mid-day whereas for most mothers in classes III, IV and V (70 per cent) it was in the evening. It was important for the whole family to sit down and eat a meal together and on weekdays this would be in the evening when the father got home.

> She has just what we have. Normally she doesn't eat breakfast. I've just started to get her to eat cereal. At playgroup she'll have biscuits and squash. Then we might go down the shops and she'll ask for some crisps or a pasty, and she'll have that or a snack at home. And then we have a proper meal in the evening. That's when we sit down together. Meat and green veg – she'll eat anything that's going.

The other main group of mothers, those from classes I and II, tended to give their children their main meal at mid-day. Few said they liked the child to eat with them. Indeed some emphasized that they disliked it.

> He doesn't eat with us much. We prefer to eat without him in the evening – because it's such chaos, and it can be late. He has his breakfast with me, after his father's left, so he has what I have then. Sometimes he has for supper what we're going to have – or he has what we had last night. Then he has his own things as well.

The impression that this mother and others gave was that feeding the child was a bit of a chore and a messy business. They looked forward to a civilized meal in the evening after the children were fed and put to bed. It seems that for some mothers socializing the child through meal-times had a rather low value. Or to put it another way, the child might be seen as having different nutritional needs from the adults – different foods and different times and intervals.

Children's diets were affected by the timing of main meals, but class was relevant too. If children had their main meal at mid-day, they had fewer sugared meals and snacks during the day than those who had their main meal in the evening, but children in class I and II households had fewer sugared meals and snacks than children in other households. Children who had their main meal in the evening had more sugared meals and snacks, irrespective of class. And those children whose mothers thought in terms of two or three main meals had fewest of all. All this is readily understandable. Children who wait till evening for their main meal will be likely to have lots of bits and pieces to keep them going through the day, and since many popular snack foods, especially drinks, are sugared, sugar is likely to be an important feature of their diet, unless their mothers are strongly opposed to it.

The data on main meals and when to have them offer some support to the thesis developed by Kerr and Charles (1984). They argue, from a study in York, that mothers think what else children eat is relatively unimportant provided they eat a 'proper' meal. So for poorer families the rest of the child's diet may be poor food. Some of the children in our study did have poor food during the day and a slap-up meal in the evening, as we have shown. But our data also show that half the mothers thought differently about meals. For them a main meal was less important than giving the child a good diet overall. The difference between the York sample and ours may be to do with the age-range of the children and position in the family. In the York study the study children ranged from 6 months to 5 years, with two-fifths aged 3 to 5, and half had elder sibs. So many were in households with established meal-times, were old enough to fit in and might be expected to fit in. Ours were all first children aged 18–36 months. With the youngest children (under-twos) mothers approved main meals, which ensured a good diet; they could enforce this because the child had limited autonomy and social life. Slightly older children (2–3 years) were old enough to make their own choices but not old enough to wait for long stretches between household main meals. The mothers were all working out their own expectations and household norms for the first time.

Social Life

Many of the 135 under-threes already had a social life that extended beyond their parents and sibs. They spent time at playgroups, with minders and nannies, visited friends and relations, and went out to restaurants. For children, as for adults, socializing includes eating and drinking. 'Yesterday', 24 per cent of the children had a meal provided by someone else – at a relative's or friend's home or at a nursery or minder's. Other children (10 per cent) had a meal at home to which a relative or friend came. Usually that meant a slightly more elaborate meal than normal, with say, a pudding or a pizza provided in honour of the guest. So a third of the children had a meal which was not provided solely as a part of the mother's provision for her household.

In addition, the children had snacks, many of them also as a part of their social life, at playgroups and round at friends' homes. And visiting friends and relatives brought little presents of food for the children. Grandmothers bring sweets as a matter of course, mothers said, wryly. Most of the snacks children had were sweetened: biscuits, sweets, chocolate, icecream and sugared drinks, and this was particularly true of gifts brought by visitors. Altogether, all but four children had something defined as a snack by their mothers 'yesterday' and most (80 per cent) had one or more sweetened snack.

What Shops Offer

What shops offer and press upon customers is crucially important in affecting food choice. Supermarkets offer large numbers of sweets, cakes, biscuits, icecreams, frozen desserts, sweetened dairy produce, sweet drinks. (At a rough estimate, such foods take up a quarter of my local supermarket's food displays.) Large supermarkets also offer plenty of fresh food, but it is a long walk past the sweetened and fatty foods to pick up the sorts of food dieticians recommend. Local shops offer a restricted range, of the most popular foods. For instance they may have only sweetened yoghurt, not unsweetened. And they tend to have little and poor quality fresh food. In the study area there was one large shopping street, situated on a busy trunk road, offering branches of most of the high street chain stores, including several large supermarkets. For some mothers, the nearest large shopping street of this kind was as much as a mile away and it was not accessible by public transport. Otherwise there were several smaller shopping streets with greengrocers, butchers, chemists, bread shops and small self-service grocery stores.

Where people shop and what they buy depends on how far they live from the shops, what transport is available and their financial resources. Busy mothers with attendant children, will choose what is most convenient. On the whole it will suit those with cars and plenty of money to go to the large supermarkets. Poorer mothers, hard-pressed with many jobs, will go to the local shops, at least on weekdays. So what foods are accessible and what resources mothers can allocate to buying food will shape their food choices.

The Daily Round

What children eat for their meals and whether they get snacks to eat and drink between-times also depends on the daily round of tasks that mothers carry out, usually with their children in attendance. Some mothers (21 per cent) said they gave their children certain meals 'yesterday' because it was quick and easy in their busy day, or because they had the food in the house (17 per cent). Doing the washing and ironing and cleaning and caring for a younger child too means less time for preparing meals. It also means stretches of time when children may be bored, fractious and seek their mothers' attention. Snacks provide children with alleviation of boredom and mothers with a respite from children's irritating demands. On expeditions to the shops, mothers kept their children going with snacks. Most of these expeditions were on foot, since few mothers had the use of a car, so they would set off armed with crisps, sweets and bottles of drink and hand these out to keep the child quiet, especially in the shops, where screaming children are unpopular.

Food and drink between meals were obviously important features of these young children's diets. Three-quarters of them had food six or more times 'yesterday'. The accounts mothers gave of their days suggest many reasons why the children had food so often and why a good deal of it was sweetened. One reason is to do with social norms. Visitors think they should give children sweets. Many of the sweet snacks were given presumably because they are easier to handle than unsweetened snacks. Playgroups gave orange squash and a biscuit half way through the session; they are less perishable and easier to store than fruit or fruit juice, and playgroup leaders know that every child will accept them. It is easier for a mother to give a child a pack of sweets to eat in her push-chair or while walking along, than to peel an orange or a banana, especially if she is in a hurry to get to the shop, or has her hands full. And there is the cost factor.

Table 6.3 *Number of sugared meals/snacks consumed 'yesterday' by mother's class (%)*

	0	1,2	3,4	5,6	7+	N
I	7	21	28	7	36	14
II	8	27	38	8	19	37
IIIa	0	23	46	8	23	26
IIIb	0	0	28	29	43	28
IV,V	4	19	23	31	23	26
N	5	24	44	22	36	131

Kendall's Tau C = .15; $p < .025$. All rows sum to 100%.

Children may waste fruit or drop it. Sweets do get eaten; and a pack of sweets is cheaper nowadays than a piece of fruit. All in all it is not surprising that snacks were firmly established as part of the children's daily diet.

The information provided by mothers also suggests reasons for the class division in the children's consumption of sugar. It was noted earlier that most children had sugar several times a day but there was a general increase in consumption along the continuum from class I to classes IV and V. One kind of explanation lies in the firmness of people's belief in the dangers of sugar to teeth, and the attempt, against all the odds, to restrict it. Among these mothers, some groups were much more likely than others to mention the dangers of sugar, and the analysis suggests that educational level as well as class were important factors. Mothers in the class groups where most had formal educational qualifications, I, II and IIIa, were very much more likely than mothers in classes IIIb, IV and V to say they tried to restrict sugar because of its effect on teeth (80 per cent against 52 per cent). And within classes IIIb, IV and V, the more highly educated mothers were much more likely to say this. This kind of explanation relies on the idea that people's actions depend heavily on their beliefs. But the data on how the children spent the day and the social contexts within which they were given food and drink suggest other pressures on behaviour which are also class related.

Well-to-do mothers probably had fewer constraints on how they spent their time than less well-off mothers. They also had more opportunity to make choices. More of them had a break while their children were looked after by someone else. They were able to carry out some jobs meanwhile. Nearly half of class I and II mothers had the use of a car during the week, so they could choose where to shop and could make other trips quickly. Compared to other mothers, they probably did not find it necessary to pacify children so often with sweets on long boring expeditions. They could also afford to be more luxurious about food – giving fruit, or nuts or fruit juice, or trying out new ideas on the child (such as cheesy biscuits, a piece of cheese, peanut butter on bread) instead of the standard child pacifiers: sweets, crisps and squash. One way or another they were able to avoid sweetened snacks more than mothers in poorer households.

It was noted earlier that in classes IIIb, IV and V children's diets deteriorated by nutritionists' standards as they got older whereas other children's did not. Discussion of factors affecting diet has pointed to possible explanations. For older children some mothers put less value on main meals; older children had entered a social setting where snacks were the norm. What children ate therefore depended on what their environment offered or pressed upon them and on how powerful mothers were in exercising choice. It is suggested that poorer mothers had less power to choose.

Obesity

Though health professionals consider obesity a health risk it was not in the forefront of mothers' minds. Only 21 per cent spontaneously raised the topic when explaining their food choices, what they aimed to provide and what they aimed to restrict. As noted above, sugary and fattening foods were an important part of the children's diets 'yesterday'. The discussion of factors affecting diet suggests that there are many pressures on mothers to give their children a fattening diet and it is a stern mother who gives her child no crisps, sweets, biscuits, sweetened drinks, chips or fried food. Many of the readily available, easy-to-eat snacks and convenience foods are sugary and fatty. They are part of the social life of young children, and busy mothers kept their children fed and happy with them, while they themselves got on with the daily tasks. In addition, mothers who favoured a family meal in the evening kept the children going during the day with quick and easy foods. Consideration of these factors suggested that they are likely to affect mothers in classes III, IV and V more than other mothers, and to push them into giving their children a more fattening diet. This was in fact the case, judging from 'yesterday's' diets.

The evidence so far suggests that most mothers did not view obesity as a health hazard for their children, or they did not think sugar and fatty foods would make them fat. However, in answer to a direct question, 'Does it matter if a child is fat?' 90 per cent (all but 14) replied that obesity was bad for a child's health, in general or specific terms. Twelve of the 14 mothers came from class III, IV and V households. Fourteen mothers is too small a number to draw conclusions from, but they did differ (in a statistically significant way) from other mothers in their patterns of health beliefs and practices.

One difference between them and other mothers was on illness causation. Most mothers thought you catch a cold from germs, bugs and viruses, but a minority (37 per cent), mainly from manual workers' classes III, IV and V, thought it was from getting cold, or from changes in temperature. The 14 mothers were more likely than others to take this more traditional view (64 per cent against 34 per cent).

Secondly, all the 14 mothers said they chose food for family custom reasons ('it's what we have, what we like'), compared to 65 per cent of other mothers. And more of them (36 per cent) gave only this sort of reason compared to 7 per cent of the rest, who mostly gave health reasons too.

Thirdly, they stood out in the way they talked about caring for their children's teeth. Whereas most other mothers (57 per cent) said they tried to restrict sugar, few of these mothers mentioned this (28 per cent).

Finally, these mothers' accounts of the children's diets 'yesterday' indicated that they gave their children rather more sugary and fatty foods. Seventy-one per cent of the 14 children compared to 46 per cent of other children, had 10 or more items of food high in sugar and/or fat.

These comparisons are suggestive rather than conclusive. They point to a possible complex of ideas about connections between food and health. Mothers' ideas about the importance of keeping warm in order to fend off colds may have included not just warm housing and plenty of clothes but a well-covered body in the other sense. Traditional patterns of eating may be particularly important among some women, and they may outweigh anything they may have heard about connections between obesity and ill health.

Discussion

Mothers' accounts of how they fed their children show there were class differences in the children's diets. A number of factors can be adduced to account for or explain these. The argument proposed here is that many factors operate to determine children's diets. Income, what shops offer, whether mothers value custom or the health-promoting virtues of food, children's preferences, the value put on main meals and when they are to be eaten, all can be seen as relevant. The evidence provided by the mothers suggests it would be foolish to argue for any of these as the crucial determinant of diet, for all are strong contenders.

But financial resources seem important, whatever other factor is in play. For instance, if you value the family eating a good main meal in the evening you may cut down on nutritious food earlier in the day, if money is tight. Similarly, if you have a busy day, you may keep the children happy with a snack, but sweets are cheaper than apples. If your day's jobs include a trip to the supermarket, again your income will determine whether you can go by car; if you walk the child may have to be pacified over long periods – again sweets are cheaper than fruit. If on the other hand you hold certain beliefs – say, about sugar's ill effects on the teeth, and if you are well off, you can afford other foods. Having a car may give you a wider choice of playgroup – some mothers chose one with apples as the mid-morning snack rather than biscuits and squash. In sum, wealth gives people freedom to make choices, including the freedom to care for their children as they wish.

Thus, financial resources affect the choices made, even where other factors are important too. However, what people believe is clearly relevant in determining the choices they make in practice, within their budget. More highly educated mothers did refer more to the kinds of knowledge that would help them make choices in line with what nutritionists recommend, notably on the ill effects of sugar on teeth.

There are implications for professionals in mothers' nutrition beliefs and practices. Some pieces of *information* could be made more available to parents. This is not to suggest that parents should be told how to behave, nor that simplistic and prescriptive messages be promoted. But if parents have reasonably full information about, for instance, the fat or sugar content of various foods, backed with evidence and argument, they can take this information into account when making decisions and choosing among priorities.

Secondly, professionals should recognize the *social context* of pressures and constraints that affect parental choices and practices. Notably, the food industry has highly sophisticated selling techniques. There is a need for professionals to add their voice to the growing demands for a national, health-conscious food policy.

Thirdly, this study has indicated *associations between poverty and poor diet*. It thus contributes to the growing evidence on the costs of child rearing and the practical effect of poverty on child-rearing practices (e.g. Burghes, 1980). Children's health is likely to suffer if they are reared on a poor diet. Health professionals must recognize the implications of poverty for child health.

Note to Chapter 6

1 We did not ask for quantities because mothers would differ in their ability to remember and because the unit of measurement (a *cup* of milk, a *bar* of chocolate, *a* salad) would conceal differences in quantity, rendering the information unreliable.

7

Caring for Children's Teeth

Introduction

As we have seen, feeding children is a centrally important feature of mothers' daily health care work. And many factors affected what the children ate. Notably, many pressures combined to ensure that they ate sugared food many times a day, even though most mothers thought sugar was bad for teeth and tried to restrict it. This chapter explores mothers' ideas about dental care in more detail. It considers how ideas about good dental status relate to those about good health status generally, as described in Chapter 5. It also considers dental care practices in the context of household routines and events. The chapter suggests that mothers vary widely in their dental care beliefs and practices. It discusses what policy measures are appropriate to help parents keep their children's teeth healthy.

Achieving Good Dental Status

What leads children to have their present state of dental health? Most mothers (61 per cent) thought that diet up to now was responsible and 40 per cent thought cleaning the teeth in various ways was an important contributory factor. In all, 79 per cent thought one or both of these kinds of management were important.

> She's got good teeth because we've got good teeth and we have a good diet and she cleans them every night.

> I give her a bit of apple to chew on and I watch her diet – I give her chocolate rather than sweets because they can be got rid of quickly, and I give her water then.
>
> Getting good teeth – it comes from the right diet. And I make him brush his teeth night and morning.

A few mothers (17 per cent) also thought their own diet before birth and during breast feeding had strengthened their babies' teeth.

> During pregnancy, I made sure I took in adequate calcium.
>
> I fed her myself, and I was careful of my diet then.

In addition, a large minority of mothers (41 per cent) thought their children's dental status depended to some extent on factors outside their present control. Mainly, they saw the character and quality of teeth as inherited (33 per cent).

> I'm not very happy with his top middle teeth. They're very close together. It tends to be in the family – his family (father's) have trouble with their middle teeth. The shape of them – it's inherited from his father's side.
>
> Both of us have good teeth, so hopefully it runs in the family.

A few (4 per cent) thought good or bad luck played a part.

> She's got excellent teeth. I don't know why – the dentist said so. I thought with all those sweets she should have bad teeth. I have good teeth myself.
>
> It's luck – and calcium in pregnancy.

And some (11 per cent) argued that all children start off with good teeth, and for these young children this natural advantage was still an important factor – as well as good care.

> I think we all have good teeth to start with.
>
> They have good teeth at this age – I've never seen a kid that age with horrible teeth, to be honest. You should teach them to brush their teeth, as well.

Thus for two-fifths of mothers non-management factors accounted at least partly for children's dental status. However, only 17 per cent argued solely in favour of non-management factors. There were no class differences on any of this.

The mothers' view that dental health in small children results at least in part from good management complements their strongly held view that good health status generally results from parental management, and parental love, but important too for some were factors that were 'given', and to that extent out of their control. Their interventionist approach explains why they thought it appropriate to care for their children's teeth 'now'; possibly the belief in 'given' factors helps to explain why dental care practices had fairly low priority in some households.

All the mothers (except one) thought dental care was appropriate now. The sorts of practices they thought good are as shown below:

Table 7.1 *Proportion of mothers who thought certain dental care practices good*

warding off	%	building up	%
brushing teeth	96	giving bone-building foods	30
restricting sugar	69	giving fluoride	22
cleaning mouth with crunchy foods	21	giving a good diet (including vitamins)	14
restricting sticky foods	13		
washing out the mouth	4		

Number of mothers = 134.

The practices suggested were of two main kinds (see Table 7.1). First were measures aimed at warding off danger: by restricting undesirable foods and by cleaning sugar and stickiness off the teeth. Second were measures aimed at building up the teeth through dietary measures to make them resistant to attack. Mothers did not differ by class as to which of these individual practices they thought important, except that fluoride (in drops, tablets or toothpaste or painted on) was favoured by 45 per cent of mothers in classes I and II, but hardly at all by any of the other mothers (6 per cent). The other major difference, discussed in Chapter 6, was that trying to restrict sugar in order to protect the teeth was mentioned by more mothers in classes I, II and IIIa than in other class groups, and educational level accounted for class differences.

All the mothers favoured warding off procedures – with tooth-brushing and sugar restriction high on the list. And 57 per cent of mothers thought one or more measure to build up teeth important; this was more likely among class I and II mothers than among other mothers (66 per cent against 46 per cent). There was a set of ideas about food and health care common among the mothers who favoured building up the teeth. They tended to refer to specifically health-directed arguments for food choice compared to other mothers, many of them gave only health-related reasons for choosing food in general; many said they chose food specifically because it was bone-building or had calcium in it and many said they tried to restrict sugar. However, within class groups there were no significant differences between the builders and the rest on these three topics. In other words the ideas were not independently related to each other, but some sets of ideas were more commonly expressed in classes I, II and to some extent in class IIIa, than in the other classes.

So people's statements about dental care were of a similar kind to their statements about food choice, and they went broadly with class. In the class groups where academic qualifications among mothers were almost universal ('O' level or above) they tended to talk more in terms of diet and fluoride as important for strengthening their children's teeth. Probably these mothers had come across publicity from the dental profession; many of them consulted baby books. Other mothers relied more on keeping children's teeth clean of sweet and sticky foods.

What Happened 'Yesterday'

Almost all mothers had carried out one or more kinds of dental care action 'yesterday' (91 per cent). The commonest action was tooth-brushing, or for the youngest children cleaning out the mouth with water or cotton wool. Sugar restriction or giving a good diet were the other main practices mentioned.

Most of the children (73 per cent) had brushed their teeth 'yesterday'. Some of the youngest children (13) had not been started off on tooth-brushing yet, according to their mothers. They had a toothbrush but it was an educational toy; 'He just plays with it'; 'he has a go sometimes, he copies us'; 'it's just to get him used to the idea'. These mothers said that at the moment the main way they looked after the children's teeth was by restricting sugary and sticky food and giving bits of apple or a drink of water. Leaving out these 13 children, 82 per cent of the rest were said to have brushed their teeth 'yesterday', or had it done for them. There were no class differences here.

But more mothers in classes I, II and IIIa said they did other things for their children's teeth as well as getting their children's teeth brushed – such as keeping down sugar and sticky things, and giving milk and fluoride and crunchy foods. This is what mothers said, and perhaps what they said shows mainly that some people attach importance to things like milk and fluoride. For, as shown earlier, while there *was* a class difference in sugar consumption 'yesterday', there was none on milk. Fluoride is in most toothpastes nowadays. So many mothers were doing things for their children even though they did not mention them.

In practice the most important difference between the class groups was on sugar. Most of the children had a lot of sugar, but there was an increase in consumption along the line from class I to classes IV and V. More important for dental health perhaps is that they tended to have fewer sugared meals and snacks, as Table 6.3 showed. So they had sugar on their teeth less often during the day.

Tooth-brushing – Who, When and Why Then?

Tooth-brushing was the principal dental care action carried out. Who did it, when and why varied widely. Major considerations were the desirability of getting the child to enjoy it and to establish the habit, and fitting it in with other household activities and routines.

Who brushed the child's teeth?

Most mothers thought they should take some part in brushing their children's teeth. Some just did it *for* the child, others took over when the child had had a go, others gave the teeth a thorough going over on some days and let the child do it otherwise. These mothers argued that their job was to teach the child and to make sure tooth-brushing was done well.

> She doesn't do it well, but she wants to do it. She wants to be involved. So she does it and then I take over.
>
> She brushes them when I remember. And if she wants to brush them she'll say, 'give me my toothbrush'. She doesn't do it properly, but she

likes the toothpaste. When we're in the bathroom, she might say, 'can I do my teeth'. And I might do it, or she might. I'm very bad on doing this, but although I've got bad habits myself, I do try and remember for her.

We clean our teeth together, him and me. After breakfast. I show him how – up and down. He has a go. He won't let me. Sometimes I do it for him to show him how.

An important consideration for mothers was the child's personality. Some children liked brushing teeth themselves. Others insisted; they resented having the job done for them. Some mothers let the child do it, to avoid battles and so that the child would enjoy tooth-brushing.

She does her teeth herself. I don't think it makes any great difference as to how her teeth are at the minute, it's just to develop the habit. I could do it for her, but if I tried it would upset her and I'm scared that would put her off.

Some mothers thought the main consideration was responsibility. ('They're her teeth, she's got to learn to do it.') Others thought the main thing was to establish a habit. ('She ought to get into the routine of doing it.') So 40 per cent of the mothers had handed over tooth-brushing to the child. Some of these also handed over the decision of when or whether tooth-brushing should happen; others thought it was up to them to suggest tooth-brushing, or remind the child. But that had to be balanced against getting the child to assume responsibility – which included remembering to brush her teeth.

He ought to do it himself. It's a good habit. So if he doesn't want to I don't force it. (*Yesterday?*) He did his teeth after lunch. He saw his toothbrush and he said 'shall I clean them', and he cleaned them. In the evening he wasn't interested in doing it. I did point out his brush to him.

There were no differences between groups of mothers in these opinions, according to class or the child's age.

When were teeth brushed and why then?

Most mothers fitted tooth-brushing in as part of the busy daily routine and specifically as part of the washing and brushing-up process (see Table 7.2). They might do it before or after a meal;

Table 7.2 *When and why children's teeth were brushed 'yesterday'*

		%
part of daily routine	– after meals	41
	– before meals	9
for efficiency	– after meals	27
when child chose		25
child doesn't brush teeth yet		10
(some mothers gave more than one reason)		

No. of mothers = 131.

that depended on when washing was done. One mother said, 'We always clean up in the morning, before breakfast, on our way downstairs.' Another, 'He has to have his breakfast, first thing, and then we go up and wash and get dressed; he does his teeth then.' In some cases children usually brushed their teeth alongside their fathers:

> His dad does his own just before he goes to work, after breakfast, so Jason does it with him. Yesterday, his dad didn't go to work, he had the day off, so Jason's teeth didn't get done.

Some mothers with an active, busy child for whom all this washing and dressing was an irrelevance to more important activities, concentrated all the cleaning up in one session:

> I do his teeth after breakfast. I'm so busy, so I catch him, and wash him and change him and clean his teeth, all in one go. It's my routine with him. And in the evening it's the same. He usually has a bottle and then I do his teeth then, last thing, after supper.

A minority of mothers (27 per cent) said that tooth-brushing took place after meals, because that was the most efficient way to clean off the food:

> He brushes his teeth after breakfast. It seems more practical then – he's more likely to enjoy brushing his teeth in the mornings. In the evenings he's beyond it. I do make sure he has a drink of water in the evening to clean his mouth out. It was after breakfast – he has such a gungy breakfast. Cereals and things. I always clean my own teeth after breakfast.

For other mothers (25 per cent) including many of those who had given the child responsibility for the job, tooth-brushing took place when the child felt like it. 'She likes doing it. She chooses when to do it. She'll pick up her toothbrush and have a go.'

Overall, 43 per cent of the children were said to have brushed their teeth once 'yesterday' and 31 per cent twice or more. Two-fifths of them brushed their teeth in the evening (25 per cent as the last thing of the day and 17 per cent followed by some more food, usually a drink). Again, class and the child's age made no difference.

> He had an apple and he brushed his teeth. It was after breakfast and after supper, while he was in the bath. Then he had his milk.

This is a mother who thinks sugar bad for teeth and tries to restrict it.

> He had a packet of sweets. And he cleaned his teeth, after his breakfast – I was taught to do it then, I think that must be why. He likes it. Sometimes he likes to do it half a dozen times a day. Then again after supper, before he went to bed. I usually give him an apple or a piece of an apple to go to bed with. And if he wakes in the night he has his orange squash because that's what he likes. He had some last night when he woke. I don't give him sweets or biscuits. They don't do much good. They're good as a treat now and then. They're full of sugar. I don't give him sugar in his tea. (*And in explaining what the child ate 'yesterday'*:) He drinks squash all through the day. He won't drink water – he hates it. I don't give him drinks at meals, because he wouldn't eat. He has his drinks any time.

The variations in tooth-brushing behaviour revealed by mothers' accounts are interesting because they suggest that it is distinctive among preventive health care practices. As with other preventive care topics, mothers had established certain kinds of practices and they readily gave reasons for what they did. But a contrast can be made in what they said about two topics: sugar and tooth-brushing. On sugar, it was clear that most mothers (86 per cent) had the same piece of knowledge: they knew sugar was bad for teeth and felt they should restrict it, though only 69 per cent said they tried to do so. So there was a generally accepted piece of knowledge, common to most mothers about the implications of behaviour for health. On tooth-brushing, they all agreed that it should take place, but they did not draw on a body of health knowledge directly as justification for their practices, so much as on tradition ('that's how I was brought up') or on the household's routines ('We wash after breakfast, when we're getting dressed'). Most did not argue that tooth-brushing at a particular time was better for the teeth.

Constraints on Dental Care 'Yesterday'

Mothers found that giving appropriate dental care was difficult in the context of daily life. The most difficult thing was to restrict sugar. As we showed in Chapter 6, though most said they tried to restrict it, there were many pressures to give sugar. Playgroups, visitors, commercial pressures, job-filled days, the children's tastes, all played a part. And as the quotation opposite shows, other child-care considerations led mothers to give sugar. Orange squash calmed the child at night. Or again:

> She cleaned her teeth after supper. I try to get the food off then. It's cleanness for the night. But then she has rose-hip to go to bed. It's sweet and sugary, but I'm not prepared not to give it to her, because it settles her down, so I weigh that against the other.

The other most important difficulty they mentioned was the children's willingness to brush their teeth. Some mothers (30) said their children *loved* brushing their teeth and all but one of these did so 'yesterday'; but of the rest, who weren't especially keen, 22 per cent did not. So the main problem was the child's refusal: 'He has to do it himself – he won't let me. Then yesterday he didn't want to do it ... so ...'

Other problems mothers mentioned were that the child was ill or tired, especially in the evening, or the mother forgot or was busy, or there was an event, an expedition or a crisis which altered the usual pattern of the day.

> We were all tired in the evening (after being out all day) and I wanted to get her off to bed, so we left it.
>
> She was a bit off colour yesterday and she slept longer than usual. So her day was different from usual.
>
> We didn't get around to it yesterday. It was washing hair day. We all washed our hair. So I didn't think about it.

Altogether, 44 per cent of the mothers equally from all class groups talked about some constraint on what they thought desirable practice, 'yesterday'.[1] In addition, analysis showed that where there was a second child in the household, the focus child was less likely to brush her teeth. Life with two under-threes is too busy for tooth-brushing.

So many factors intervene to affect dental care. Mothers have to juggle people's needs and wishes, their own commitments, and cope with emergencies and changes to routine daily life. Compared to these dental care may lack urgency and importance. Other health needs of adults and children in the household may make it appropriate to shelve the child's dental care.

Help with Dental Care from Professionals

Mothers of young children are mostly in frequent touch with doctors and health visitors for illness and developmental checks, and their knowledge and practices may be modified by these contacts. Dental care knowledge and practices seemed to be heavily shaped by individual personality and approaches and by domestic circumstances and traditions. So it was interesting to explore contacts with health professionals about children's dental health.

Most of the mothers (79 per cent) thought their children's teeth were good: 'They're straight and white'; 'they do the job pretty well'; or 'lovely'; or even 'like pearls' or 'fabulous – they look perfect to me'. A few said the child had one or more crooked teeth. But 19 of the 135 mothers (14 per cent) said their children had already had dental problems – with 'yellow' or 'black' spots or patches, damaged or lost teeth. A high proportion of these 19 children (9) were in class IV and V households.[2] Eleven of these 19 children had been to the dentist, equally from the different class groups.

The other kind of dental problem children had was with teething; 38 per cent were said to have had teething problems at some point in their lifetime. In the last three months, 26 children had had one or more episodes of illness with a group of symptoms which led mothers to say the child was teething: symptoms such as teething, red cheeks and ears, temperature, runny nose, diarrhoea (see also Chapter 8). In few of these cases (7) did mothers consult a doctor (none consulted a health visitor or a dentist) and then only if they were uncertain about the diagnosis (5 mothers), or worried by the high level of the child's distress (2 mothers). Some talked it over with friends and relatives. Most were not worried by the episode and the reasoning was that teething even when painful was a normal part of development, and so nothing to worry about. A doctor confirmed this view for one mother:

> His cheeks went bright red, and he got very hot and he went to bed about 10 and then woke up and he was very whiny. I took his temperature; it was 102°. We rang the doctor at about 10.00 and meanwhile I just gave him a junior aspirin. His breathing gets very fast and the rate of his heart beat gets so fast, that's what's really worrying. The doctor said he had a clear chest, no soreness or swelling in his throat. He said, 'It's probably just his teeth. I won't give him anything as there's nothing wrong with him'.

So mothers did not always seek advice for dental problems, and for some, teething was normal and so not worrying. However, almost all of them (93 per cent) thought children should go to a dentist for check-ups and most (77 per cent) thought they should go before the age of three. There was no class difference on this.

> I'd like Jane to go now, when she's about three. To make sure her teeth are alright. So she can learn to look after her teeth. Before she has to go in pain. It's better for her to go before that, so she knows you don't have to be in pain to go to the dentist. I don't like them. I only go if I get toothache.

The minority view (13 per cent) was that young children do not need to go if there is nothing wrong, and that school-age children will be routinely seen by school dentists.

> She doesn't need to go to the dentist yet. I don't mind if they check her over at school. But there's no need yet. Her teeth are alright. When she goes to school (at 5) she'll be checked there.

And four mothers took the even more traditional view that a visit to the dentist was appropriate only if you were in pain.

Where did mothers get the idea that children should go to the dentist to be checked? One source of knowledge must be the local network of mothers exchanging notes, possibly reinforced by advice in baby books. In the study area the District Health Authority (DHA) gives its view, by sending out a letter to mothers of two-and-a-half year olds, suggesting they bring the child to one of the health authority dental clinics. Half the mothers of two-and-a-half year olds (53 per cent) said they had had a card from the DHA, but a much higher proportion of mothers in classes I, II and IIIa mentioned it, than of other mothers. There may have been a class difference in whether mothers received the card, since there was high mobility among families in classes IV and V in the last year, so in some cases the DHA might not have caught up with them. But probably some mothers did not remember the card, or it was not at the forefront of their minds when talking to us. Many mothers especially in classes III, IV and V had stressful lives – the arrival of a card from the DHA may not have been a notable event.

But was it easy for mothers to go to the dentist? The local Regional Health Authority (RHA) is well provided with dentists by national standards, and the area of the study especially well provided, according to the RHA Strategic Plan, 1978–88. Community dental services are provided at health centres for school children and in some cases for under-fives. In the study area, the two health centres had each a dental service for under-fives. Several mothers said they were pleased there was a service specially for children, readily available at the clinic.

> I'm pleased he can go up the clinic. I never went when I was young and my teeth are bad now. They can watch his teeth, now while he's young.

Those who had taken their child to the clinic dentist all said the visit went well, and for many it was a contrast with their own memories of childhood visits to the dentist.

Some mothers (27 per cent) said they were deterred by fear of the dentist from having professional care themselves, and this was more common in classes IIIb, IV and V. Thirty-nine per cent of the mothers had not been to the dentist in the last year with higher proportions in classes IV and V (61 per cent). Mothers said they hated going, or that they were too busy. Some commented that it was expensive, and that they had last been in pregnancy when it was free. It is interesting that mothers felt they should go to the dentist regularly, though it is not clear whether they saw this as a social norm, or as a means to good dental health. However this may be, the fact that they were afraid themselves made them all the more determined that their children should start early before they were in pain, so that they did not develop this fear.

> I went myself this week. I go every six months. It's booked in advance to make me go. You have to pay even if you don't turn up. I get into a

panic. I really shake. It makes me physically sick. I have to make myself go. It's the noise that gets me. So I have to take her, so she won't be frightened. At about two, two-and-a-half.

I went myself two-and-a-half years ago. I'm terrified. I bit a dentist's hand once as a child. He told me to go away and not come back. Then I had the school dentist. They gave me a cocaine injection that didn't work. I have to be knocked out for a filling. So he's going to go, and he's not going to be afraid. My husband's going to take him. They should go when they've got some teeth. By age two anyway.

It seems mothers thought they should take the child to the dentist, so she would be used to it before repair work had to be done. However, very few suggested, like Jane's mother quoted above, that the dentist might teach the child how to care for her teeth. Dental decay was seen as inevitable, and the visit to the dentist was for repair work, not for preventing problems.

Finally, a quarter of the mothers (24 per cent) said they had taken their children for a dental check-up. The proportion declined from 33 per cent in class I to 11 per cent in classes IV and V. Some of the mothers who had a dentist they trusted had taken the child along when they had an appointment themselves; others went to the health centre clinic. Mothers obviously felt it was an event to be carefully planned and handled. Some took the child first of all so she could watch them behaving cheerfully in the dentist's chair. Others talked to the child about it in advance, or played at dentists:

She brushes them with my husband. They play at dentists. He's concerned about teeth, including his own. She's been playing at having her teeth examined.

Other mothers thought they should wait till the child was older, better able to cope. Their knowledge of the child was the guide:

You should take them to the dentist by the age of three. But I won't take him because I know he won't cooperate. I know because of taking him to the doctor and the shoe-shop. He wouldn't go to the dentist to be poked about. So I'll leave it till I go at Easter and he'll just go with me then. Then I'll take him when he's about four to be seen himself.

Discussion

There were no class differences in approaches to dental care, nor in rates of tooth-brushing 'yesterday'. But socially advantaged mothers were more likely to favour building up teeth and managed to give less sugar 'yesterday' and they tended to favour a diet that would help to strengthen the child's body. To the extent that diet affects dental status, their children had a better chance than others. Reasons for class differences in sugar consumption were discussed in Chapter 6. The children from socially advantaged backgrounds also seemed more likely to establish the habit of going to the dentist than others. This may be because more of the mothers went themselves, fewer feared the dentist and more remembered that the DHA had offered an appointment for the child. In practice, more of the children had been for a preventive check.

Class differences in adults' preventive behaviour for themselves were not a focus of this study but possible explanations for these differences in mothers' use of dentists can be suggested. Use of services by socially disadvantaged mothers was probably difficult – both in their childhood and now. Some of the mothers' bad childhood experiences of dentists may have been due to area variation in quality and quantity of services, with socially disadvantaged areas having worse services. Mobility probably made it more difficult to find and keep a good dentist. Living in stressful circumstances deterred people from making the effort to use the preventive dental service. Dental care fees under the NHS were almost certainly a deterrent.[3]

Mothers saw management practices by parents as essential for children's good dental health status. And they all said they were carrying out various practices 'now', mainly restricting sugar and brushing the teeth. It also seemed that they saw a role for professional help, mainly to repair teeth, so they wanted their children to get used to going to the dentist.

Two points stood out as regards practices. First, practices were affected by many intervening events and pressures in daily life, and actions designed specifically to protect teeth seemed to have fairly low priority. Secondly, there was wide variation in practices and views on tooth-brushing. Perhaps dental care is pushed aside on some days because it is not something that gets immediate, observable results in improving or maintaining the child's health. And mothers may view the preservation of good teeth as well-nigh impossible; the data suggest that many mothers viewed dental decay as inevitable. But these two points also suggest that mothers did not have access to a firm, consistent body of knowledge about what was appropriate and important in dental care. This may be at least in part because there appear to be various messages beamed at mothers, from the dental professions and from baby books.

What does the dental profession recommend? A policy document, reporting on a seminar of top dentists, proposes three main strategies (HEC, 1978). First, people should aim to reduce sugar intake and should try to restrict sugared foods to mealtimes. Non-sugared snacks between meals have little adverse effect on the teeth. Secondly, they should clean their teeth thoroughly at least once a day to clean off plaque, in order to prevent periodontal disease. They should use fluoride toothpaste. Brushing in itself has little effect on dental decay, but the fluoride strengthens the teeth. Thirdly, they should press for the fluoridation of water supplies and meanwhile give their children flouride drops or tablets. This message is enclosed in a leaflet aimed at parents. The report argues that general diet has no proven effect on dental decay (see also Davis, 1980). The report is a formal statement not readily accessible to the public. But a pamphlet available at the same time and directed at parents argues that a balanced diet of protein, carbohydrate, vitamins, phosphorous and calcium is important for teeth building. This view is also promoted by two popular baby books (Jolly, 1981; Leach, 1979). These authors also say parents should take their children to the dentist by the age of two – more ambitious advice than that of the British Dental Association which recommends a visit before children start school.[4]

Probably mothers have varied ideas about dental care for children and do not give it high priority partly because they do not hear professional views on it, or hear conflicting messages. Health professionals may themselves hold varying views and may or may not offer dental advice to mothers. It is not clear whether health visitors routinely offer advice to mothers specifically on dental care, but it has been suggested (Williams and Fairpo, 1984) that they lack knowledge that accords with the views of the dental profession, so if they do advise mothers this may add to confusion and to variation in practices. GPs, whom mothers tend to see often, probably steer clear of advising mothers about dental care, which they see as another profession's province. Mothers, like other adults, go infrequently to the dentist themselves and probably few dentists offer advice about preventive care for young children, and especially not to an adult attending without a child. In addition, given the nature of the service offered, most people probably see the dentist as a curer not a preventer, and may not ask for, or respect, preventive advice. For most people, the dentist is a more remote figure than the doctor; contacts are fewer and so are discussions about dental care.

The foregoing does not imply that it is necessarily a good thing for people's health care of their children to be heavily conditioned by what professionals say. But, while children's dental health has improved over the last ten years, there is still room for further improvement (c.f. Todd and Todd, 1985, chs 4 and 7). And the data do suggest that many mothers would find it useful to discuss dental care with a professional and that they need clear consistent messages. It was also clear that mothers started caring for children's teeth early on – the youngest children were 18 months old, and mothers thought diet was important from birth. So mothers might welcome the chance to discuss dental care when the child is a baby or toddler. From the professionals' point of view, it would seem useful to start getting messages across as early as possible, and both parents and professionals stand to benefit from increasing their understanding of one another's perspectives on dental care.

At a more general level, the mothers' accounts of dental care suggests that though they were concerned about their children's dental status, there were many factors that inhibited dental care in practice. It seems unreasonable to put all the onus on mothers (or even on parents); to expect individuals to improve the nation's dental health, each one single-handed against the mighty pressures of the food industry, established social customs and the complexities of family life (c.f. Cowell and Sheiham, 1981). As with safety care, where, if we want fewer accidents, the best course is probably to improve the children's environment, so with dental care. It is already clear that the introduction of fluoride in water and toothpaste and measures to decrease the sugar content of some foods have had beneficial effects on children's teeth.

Notes to Chapter 7

1 There were no class differences in the number of mothers who mentioned constraints on dental care 'yesterday', and the numbers

giving each type of constraint are too small to analyse by class, or child's age.
2 The 19 children with dental problems so far, by class: I 2; II 2; IIIa 3; IIIb 3; IV and V 9.
3 Blaxter and Paterson (1982) Chapter 9 note the scarcity of dentists in a poor area of Aberdeen; Lobstein and Sheiham (1980) found that Community Health Councils especially in London areas found high rates of concern among people about *finding a dentist* and about *charges* at dentists.
4 HEC leaflets are usually not dated. The ones referred to were available in clinics at the time we did our interviewing (1982). The one recommending that parents pressurize local authorities and MPs for fluoridation is called 'Is this what you want for your child?' The one on diet is called 'Diet and Healthy Teeth'. The one recommending a visit to the dentist before school-age is titled 'The Six-Year Molars'.

SECTION C

Coping with Illness at Home

8

Caring for Ill Children

Introduction

An important part of mothers' health care work is the care of ill children. Most of this takes place at home, out of the public eye, and only a minority of illness episodes are seen by health professionals. We explored the kinds of knowledge mothers brought to the observation of their children, diagnosis of illness, and care. Their detailed knowledge of the child's history and resistance was particularly important in this work. And their accounts also show the importance of the domestic context in shaping and constraining the care of ill children. This chapter suggests that health professionals to whom mothers turn for help, will be best placed to give help if they recognize and build on mothers' knowledge, and if they take domestic circumstances into account when discussing conditions with mothers.

Symptoms and Episodes

We started by asking the 135 mothers to describe anything unusual they had noticed in their child (the focus child) recently, firstly 'yesterday', then going back over the last few weeks, and up to three months ago. To help recall we read out a list of 15 symptoms, which we had found in extensive pilot interviews to be the ones most commonly noticed by mothers (see Table 8.1). In the event, over 80 per cent of the episodes recounted took place within the last month, but we included the rest to make up numbers. Once the mother had started talking about the

Table 8.1 *Frequency with which mothers associated certain symptoms with specific categories of illness (%)*

		Diagnoses					
Symptoms	No. of mentions	Respiratory/ENT %	Gastric %	Skin %	Teething %	No diagnosis %	Other N
Appetite	124	9	22	13	10	15	(8)
Energy	163	12	13	6	10	12	(54)
Clinging	86	8	4	2	8	8	(20)
Pain	85	7	6	6	9	6	(16)
Vomiting	53	3	15	0	1	4	(18)
Diarrhoea	50	1	20	2	6	2	(8)
Runny nose	129	19	.8	.9	11	8	(12)
Cough	86	13	0	2	10	6	(3)
Appearance	86	7	2	9	7	7	(20)
Mood/behaviour	67	4	2	7	6	7	(19)
Inflammation	51	2	.8	11	10	4	(10)
Temperature	83	7	7	6	5	10	(16)
Rash	55	.4	0	35	2	3	(9)
Breathing problems	43	5	4	.9	4	4	(1)
Other	39	3	2	4	4	3	(12)
Total N	1,200	492	118	115	104	145	226

All columns sum to 100%. No. of mothers = 135.

occurrence of symptoms she usually then went on to describe the progress of the episode: what happened, how the child looked, what was problematic, what decisions were made, what relatives, friends and the doctor said, what care and treatment were given. In order to collect information systematically we had a list of prompts on these topics, to supplement the mothers' accounts.

Of the 15 symptoms listed, the most commonly reported by mothers were changes in energy level, runny noses and loss of appetite. Coughs, changes in appearance (e.g. pallor, puffy eyes), clinging behaviour, aches and pains, and temperatures were also common (see Table 8.1, first column). We asked mothers what they thought the episode was and in most cases they gave a diagnosis.

Altogether the children had 350 conditions between them.[1] The most common were respiratory – colds, tonsillitis (including sore throats, and throat infections) and ear conditions (143). There were 61 gastro-intestinal problems, 41 skin conditions, 36 teething episodes, 4 infectious diseases of childhood, and 6 genito-urinary conditions. Twenty-three conditions were not diagnosed, 8 were given the name virus, bug or germ, 8 more thought not to be illness. There were 13 other conditions (the complete list of conditions is given in the Appendix Table A.12).

Class Differences in Illness

Judging by their mothers' accounts, a quarter of the 135 children (27 per cent) had what we have termed 'persistent conditions'. These conditions had all lasted for more than three months and included recurring or constant respiratory infections often dating from a serious illness during the first year of life, a few congenital conditions mentioned by the mother as a continuing source of vulnerability in their child, and chronic eczema. We refer to these conditions as persistent rather than chronic in that they include both constant and recurring conditions, and because they occurred to children perceived by their mothers to be more fragile and to need a different form of health care compared with other children.

There were no differences by class in the reported overall incidence of acute episodes of illness, or in the number of days of acute illness during the last three months, when class was controlled by the age and sex of the child and by the season in which episodes occurred. That is, *younger* children and *boys* had more episodes and children had more episodes in *winter* months than in summer ones. There was, however, a broad class division in the proportions of children who had persistent conditions, with 34 per cent in classes III, IV and V, compared to 18 per cent in classes I and II. The age and sex of the children made no difference to this. It was notable that much of the class difference is accounted for by persistent respiratory conditions – 21 per cent of class III, IV and V children had these, compared to 5 per cent of class I and II children. Not surprisingly, the persistently ill children had very many more episodes of acute illness in the last three months than other children; twice as many had three or more episodes (76 per cent compared to 38 per cent of other children).

Among the 135 households, occupational class and material disadvantage went closely together. Nevertheless, within class groups, some households were worse off than others, and analysis of some key variables representing material disadvantage (no garden, no telephone) set against persistent illness showed that within classes III, IV and V, persistently ill children were likely to come from the more disadvantaged households.

In sum, there were some households (27 per cent) with a child who had a distinct pattern of illness and was more ill than the rest of the focus children. These children tended to belong to relatively disadvantaged families in classes III, IV and V.

Mothers' Knowledge of Children's Illness

Diagnosis

The interview data allowed us to approach mothers' knowledge of illness in several ways. To begin with it was useful simply to examine the way they associated symptoms with specific categories of illness. Table 8.1 shows this. The categories consist of our summary of the diagnostic labels mothers put on their children's illnesses.

We should note initially that not all the remembered episodes were considered to be illness. For instance mothers said: 'She wasn't ill – it was just a runny nose', or 'She just wasn't hungry yesterday, otherwise she was alright'.

As might be expected, mothers associated runny noses and coughs most frequently with respiratory diagnoses, but they quite frequently put runny noses down to teething. Similarly, mothers associated vomiting and diarrhoea most frequently with alimentary and gastric diagnoses, but they sometimes saw diarrhoea as an accompaniment of teething. They associated rashes overwhelmingly with skin diagnoses.

Teething and associated discomfort among children in our age group may have been linked by mothers with the eruption of the molars around the age of two, a process which may last for a number of weeks or even months. Mothers seemed to be undisturbed by the wide variety of symptoms they associated with teething, which they considered a natural phase in the child's development. For 80 per cent of reported episodes of teething mothers did not contact a doctor. So there was a risk that children with symptoms indicating another, more serious condition could have had inappropriate care.

Mothers' accounts of what symptoms caused them to think their children were ill, when set against their accounts of what a healthy child is like, indicate that they judged the onset of illness by evidence of a falling away from such characteristics of good health as they observed as usual in their child: normal appetite, normal activity levels and certain amounts of sleep at certain intervals. Changes in energy levels and appetite were two of the three symptoms most commonly observed – along with runny noses – which led mothers to keep a close eye on the child and to think there might be something wrong (c.f. Cunningham-Burley, 1984). So the symptoms mothers noticed most, or remembered most often, were behavioural symptoms, rather than indications of physical change or disturbance. These came second in importance: various evidences of pain, cough and temperature, changes in appearance, especially facial appearance, as well as other behavioural changes, such as becoming more clinging than usual.

Changes in appetite, energy and temperature seemed to give mothers the least good help towards deciding what if anything was wrong with their child, in that where one of these symptoms occurred mothers often did not offer a specific diagnosis of the condition. Changes in appetite and energy were often the first symptoms of a child's illness, before anything specific happened (like pain or spots). Temperature change is common in young children and as mothers noted, can signal anything from excitement to a serious illness. Appetite, energy, and temperature changes were all symptoms worth watching because they *might* herald illness which would involve other symptoms too – or they might not. Other more specific symptoms were more likely to lead mothers to think their child was ill, and to make a diagnosis.

Some mothers did not give a name to the episode, others gave as a name or diagnosis, the dominant symptom, such as 'runny nose', or 'diarrhoea'; others gave a label, such as tonsillitis, measles, ear infection. Mothers' diagnoses differed from those of doctors. Seventy-three per cent of mothers who consulted a GP had made a different diagnosis or received no confirmation of their own diagnosis or they did not reach a diagnosis before consulting the doctor. Seventeen per cent of mothers were told by their GP that their child's condition was more serious than they thought and this was more common among mothers from classes

I and II than among other mothers; however, when the mothers' 'wrong diagnoses' and 'no diagnoses' were added together the class difference disappeared. In other words mothers from classes I and II were more willing to suggest a diagnosis (though they were sometimes 'wrong') than mothers from classes III, IV and V.

Causes

What did they think caused the illnesses in their children? The main causes proposed were germs, bugs, viruses and infections. Fifty-nine per cent of mothers advanced some version of *germ theory* as a cause of one or more recent illness. This was much commoner among class I and II mothers than among other mothers (76 per cent against 47 per cent).

> Flu – she picks up things very quickly at school. If there's a bug going round, most of the children get it. She passes them in the corridor and the bugs are floating around and she catches it.
>
> He's had a runny nose and a cough. His cousin had it and he was in constant contact with him.
>
> She had a cold. I talked to my Mum, she said keep her warm. My Dad said she hadn't been kept warm. I said you don't get a cold like that – it's a germ.

A smaller proportion of mothers, 18 per cent, thought the child's illness was caused by eating something specific. The food was either bad, or it did not agree with the child.

> She was sick a week ago. It was something she was eating.
>
> Diarrhoea – it was brought on by fruit.

Changes in the weather or temperature, or the effects on the child of a spell of very cold or very hot weather were also popular causes. Thirty-five per cent of mothers advanced such thermal reasons for illness once or more. There were no clear patterns by class on this, except that much higher proportions of mothers in classes IV and V (58 per cent) gave *thermal reasons*.

> He's had a cold. He gets it when we go to Scotland – it's a cold house there, no central heating, draughty.
>
> He had diarrhoea for two days. He was sick twice in the day. It was in the hot weather – it was that brought it on.
>
> Cold – she was playing outside without a coat, and playing with water in the bathroom.

For some mothers more than one factor was responsible.

> She had a cold – she caught it off someone, or it could have been the teething. I think it was brought on by the weather, and change of place. We'd come back from Wales the weekend before, and that may have affected her.

> He had a cold... A lot of my friends' children had colds, he got it from them, I expect. And they tend to get more colds in the winter.

As noted above, many mothers, equally from all classes, put conditions that included symptoms such as diarrhoea, sore throats and fever down to *teething* (28 per cent).

> She was going to get her new tooth – her gum swelled and she always gets a runny nose or a cough. She had the runny nose for two weeks and the cough for a day, but the tooth never showed.

Stress on the child was seen as a contributing factor by some mothers (28 per cent), equally from all classes. Along with other factors stress pushed the child over the edge into illness.

> She was sick in the car. She may be going through a phase – she doesn't like going in the car. And it was very hot, and she's on the antibiotics as well – they have a general effect on her.

Finally, 26 per cent argued that the child's health pattern in the past, or her *physical predisposition* was a cause of an episode of illness. This was much commoner among mothers in classes III, IV and V than among other mothers (34 per cent against 14 per cent) because many of them had children with chronic or recurrent conditions, and they thought their children were vulnerable both to these and to other conditions, such as colds.

> He had a cold, with the wheezing. He's had the chest infection before. He does get that.

> It was her eczema flaring up again.

> She's a bit chesty. It tends to go to her chest.

> She got this build-up of wax. She gets that.

> Earache. She keeps getting it. When her glands swelled up I thought she was getting another attack. The doctor said she'd probably get it again.

The 'lay referral network' as a source of knowledge

The mothers were first-time mothers, learning on the job. By now, with the child through her first eighteen months or more, they had built up a good deal of knowledge from experience, though as noted earlier, some still faced the unfamiliar – such as high temperatures, and then they tended to contact the doctor. But many nursed their children through minor illness without contacting the doctor. They altered the child's diet, gave her more opportunity to sleep, kept her warm, or cool, cuddled her, sat with her, cleaned her up. They also treated the child with medicines and tonics.

Knowledge of what to do came partly in response to the child's need, from experience of what seemed to work, from talking with friends and relations and from baby books. Nearly half the mothers (47 per cent) had turned to a friend or relative in the last three months to discuss the child's illness.

This advice was useful in a number of ways. It provided *information*, for instance that this condition was common at this age, at this time of year or currently in the neighbourhood.

> They get a lot of colds at this age.
>
> My friends all said their children had had the same thing.
>
> My sister said her children had all had this deafness in the winter time.

Friends and relatives gave *diagnoses*, which often set a mother's mind at rest ('My sister said it was conjunctivitis and to bathe it in cold water.' 'We'd been with my sister and her daughter had the mumps. She thought Sandra had it too.')

They offered *advice* on nursing, based on their own experience, and they gave the names of useful remedies.

> I talked to my mother, and she said make her drink as much as possible.
>
> My friend said she had too many fats in her diet.
>
> My sister said aspirin usually helped.
>
> I talked to friends and they said, 'Have you tried Bonjela?' I did get some, but I didn't use it.

Some said, take him to the *doctor*. This was common among mothers' own mothers. 'I mentioned it (*diarrhoea*) to my Mum and she said, 'Have you spoken to the doctor?'' Probably these older women did not wish to be cast as know-alls, and they did want to pay tribute to their daughter's responsibility for the child (c.f. Blaxter and Paterson, 1982, ch. 15).

The lay advice and information gave mothers both support and a range of options to consider in deciding what to do to help the child. At each episode of illness mothers who had good support from friends and relatives were able to add to their store of knowledge and acquire more confidence in caring for the child. There was a broad divide by class in mothers' use of this kind of help. Mothers in classes I and II were more likely than other mothers to say they nursed their child using advice from friends or relatives and they were also more likely than others to say they used their own judgement. And more of them gave as a reason for not contacting the doctor that the illness was 'not serious enough' or 'just a cold'. So these mothers, few of whom had persistently ill children, were relying on and building on their own and other lay opinion as a basis for action. They were also much more likely to say they had turned to a book for advice. The mothers in classes III, IV and V were much more likely to rely on the doctor's advice, when deciding what nursing and what treatments to give. Probably this broad pattern of difference results from the fact that more of them had persistently ill children who were 'under the doctor'. In addition some did not have enough people to turn to. It is worth noting in this connection that only 38 per cent of those with an unsatisfactory social network said they consulted friends/relatives in the last three months about specific symptoms, compared to 56 per cent of the rest.

Mothers' Care of Ill Children

For over half the episodes reported (59 per cent) mothers cared for the child without consulting a health professional. Many of these episodes were of symptoms or conditions familiar to the mother and she knew how to deal with them. Some were trivial ('just a runny nose', 'she was off her food'), and the mother was not worried.

(*Diarrhoea*) I just changed his nappy more, to stop him getting a sore bottom.

(*Chesty cold*) I made sure she was wrapped up warmly. I gave her a lot to drink – Lucozade, orange juice, water.

(*Earache*) I had a look and it was all waxed up and it had gone hard so I softened it up and cleaned it all out with warm water and cotton buds. And then it settled down.

(*Teething*) I cuddled him more and gave him biscuits.

(*Cold*) I gave him a junior Disprin and some baby cough mixture and rubbed him with Vick. And I went up in the evening to see him more often than usual.

Mothers dealt with minor conditions by changing management as regards diet, rest, temperature and hygiene. They gave the child more or less or different food, extra drinks or treats to cheer her up. They gave more opportunity to sleep, sometimes moving the child onto a sofa near at hand so the child was part of the social scene and could be talked to and watched for changes. They kept children warm by wrapping them up and keeping them indoors, or cooled them down by sponging them and reducing the amount of clothing or bedding. They paid more attention to hygiene than usual – cleaning the child and giving extra baths and washing her (and themselves) more. They also gave medicaments from the chemist or left over from previous episodes. Popular ones were Calpol, junior aspirin, various cough mixtures, zinc and castor oil cream.

Common threads that emerge from mothers' accounts are that once the child had a symptom they gave her extra attention and time. They monitored her closely for other symptoms, for deterioration and improvement. They nursed the child using methods that had worked in the past. During the acute phase they kept the child close at hand, partly to offer comfort and love as a means of curing the child, but also to keep an eye on her condition.

(*Bronchitis*) I sponged him down. And I made more of a fuss of him generally. I took him into bed with me, 'cos he couldn't sleep.

(*Teething*) We fetched him into bed with us and cuddled him to sleep.

(*Measles*) I made sure she had lots of drinks. Bathed her face with cotton wool and boiled water. And I just held her most of the time.

(*Stomach upset*) I gave him a hot water bottle. And lots of fluids. I got him off to bed early and I went in to see him a couple of times in the night.

These methods of caring for ill children seemed to be common currency among mothers. We did not discern any class differences. While mothers' use of lay advice did show class differences, the basic methods – mainly tried and tested commonsense plus careful loving attention to detail – did not.

However, mothers also have to decide whether and when to consult professionals for their children. Study of mothers' accounts indicated that a number of factors were important, but first we looked to see if any mothers were deterred from using the services. Other studies have suggested that some mothers, especially those from socially disadvantaged households, are deterred from contacting the doctor because of their perceptions of the characteristics of the service or out of deference (c.f. Blaxter and Paterson's (1982) study of older women). But, only a small number of our mothers (9 or 6 per cent), equally from all social classes, commented that they were deterred because the advice offered was generally poor (3), because they did not want to bother the doctor (2) or because the surgery was shut (4).

In addition, 30 per cent of mothers, equally from all classes, said they had difficulty deciding whether the condition merited professional advice. There were a number of variations on this theme. Some mothers wanted a diagnosis, especially if they thought it could be one of two or three conditions, yet they were not sure it was serious enough to be worth finding out, or the doctor might not be correct. Some mothers were uncertain what the condition was and whether medical intervention could help it. Others thought it was a minor, self-righting condition, but then after a week or so wondered if it needed medicine to clear it up. Others were uncertain which professional to consult – the health visitor or the doctor; the GP or the hospital.

This mother deliberated, and opted against contacting the doctor, once she and the father had decided what it was and the child seemed better.

> I took him out on the toboggan. He was well wrapped up. Then next day he woke up and he had a runny nose. I was wondering whether it was a cold or whether he got so cold on his face that it was his sinuses. The mucous coming down was white. There was no yellow. His hair went very fine and wispy. I checked his throat with a teaspoon. I was worried by the runny nose. I always think it's going to turn into something worse. So I wasn't sure whether to go to the doctor. And we kept on taking his temperature. It was completely normal. So we waited a few hours more and then he got up and he was playing with the dog and we agreed it was a little cold. So we didn't contact the doctor because he'd just perked up again.

This next mother decided eventually that the condition was serious enough to warrant a trip to the doctor.

> His appetite was affected, for about a fortnight, and he was definitely a bit low on energy. His throat hurt and he had vomiting and

diarrhoea. And he looked poorly. Rather big under the eyes. Pale and he lost weight. He looked thinner. And he needed fussing over. I was worried about him one evening for a time. I wondered if I ought to take him to the doctor. It was my ignorance, really. I'd know another time. Because I couldn't decide if it was his throat that was hurting him or his stomach. Since then I've looked it up in my baby book and it says that glands in the stomach sometimes swell with tonsillitis. So I should have known better, but that was basically it. He was holding his stomach, yet he wouldn't take any liquid. He was being almost hysterical. Eventually I got him to take something. It was that confusion of not knowing how to diagnose it. I think he'd had it for about a week before. And this in itself is a dilemma. Do I as soon as I think it's coming take him off to the doctor, on suspicion? And yet I'm not that keen to pump him full of things. Or do I wait till he's got it and then take him, and it'll take that much longer to get over it . . .? It wasn't till he was sick (*vomiting*) that I thought, oh, come on, this is really something, he's got something. I must get some medical advice. (*Child diagnosed by doctor as having tonsillitis.*)

The mothers' dilemmas seem to have a common feature. They could not decide, using the various pieces of knowledge they had, what was the best course of action. They were uncertain what symptoms suggest what condition, whether medical intervention could help and what kind of help to use. The mothers' stories also demonstrate that they were fully aware that in many cases illness is self-limiting and that the doctor can do little to help the course of nature. Some also disliked giving their children medicines and especially antibiotics.

Why mothers contacted the doctor?

If mothers wanted help with ill children from a professional, it was mainly the GP they turned to. In the last 3 months 72 per cent had contacted the GP, 15 per cent the health visitor, 3 per cent the chemist, and 19 per cent had taken the child to hospital.

In Chapter 9, mothers' accounts of consultations with doctors are described in order to consider what they hoped to get from the doctor. Here we look at some factors that seemed to lead mothers to consult the doctor: certain symptoms, persistent illness, and poor social support.

Worry
We thought initially that mothers might divide into groups according to whether worry about symptoms did or did not lead them to contact the doctor, but this was not so. When mothers reported worrying they almost always said they contacted the doctor. This could be a function of story-telling. While ordering the episode and making sense of it in the telling, people may see worry as a factor justifying contact. However, where children were ill on the interview day, and mothers were weighing up what to do 'now' (rather than constructing a story for the interviewer) they also tended to say that they might go to the doctor 'because they were worried'. As noted earlier, there was little evidence of deference inhibiting service use. So if there were children not taken to the doctor for serious conditions needing medical help – though on the face of it this seems unlikely, from mothers' accounts – then this would be only if the mothers were neglecting the children (also unlikely) or did not know the seriousness of a set of symptoms.

Symptoms
Some symptoms led to contact with the doctor more than other symptoms. Contact with the doctor was reported most frequently for children with temperatures, coughs and aches and pains and least frequently for children with diarrhoea, energy change, difficult behaviour and change of mood. There were no class differences in the frequency with which mothers reported contacting the doctor for various symptoms.

It seemed possible that mothers who noticed a symptom for the first time might be especially worried and uncertain and so would be particularly likely to contact their GP. In fact most mothers had seen most of the symptoms before, but mothers faced with unfamiliar rashes and aches and pains (including sore throats and earache) were more likely to contact the doctor than mothers whose children had had them before. Mothers quite often seemed uncertain about diagnosing sore throats and ear infections, possibly because the site of discomfort was inside the body and difficult to see.

Persistent conditions
There were class differences in how often mothers said they had contacted the doctor in the last three months. Two factors

accounted for these differences: persistent conditions in the children, and poor social support. These factors suggested reasons why some mothers felt they needed frequent professional help in caring for their ill children.

Mothers in classes III, IV and V reported contacting the doctor more frequently than mothers in classes I and II, but when consultation rates were controlled according to whether the child had a persistent illness, the class difference disappeared. However, among mothers of persistently ill children, those in classes III, IV and V said they consulted more frequently than those in classes I and II. Perhaps this was because more of them had children with persistent respiratory conditions and they needed professional help and discussion for these conditions more often than mothers did for skin conditions (the other main kind of persistent condition).

Mothers of persistently ill children may have consulted the doctor more partly because they had distinctive perceptions of their children's health and concern about an episode compared to other mothers. They were concerned not just about the symptoms and outcome of a particular episode of illness, but about the child's health status overall. They tended – very much more than other mothers – to think their children had poor resistance to illness. Indeed only 18 per cent of mothers with a persistently ill child thought she was more resistant to illness than other children, compared to 50 per cent of other mothers.

> She's allergic to picking things up. I don't know why. But she does.
> He's prone to things. He was born with a weakness.
> She does fall ill easy, easier than the baby. Things just seem to come upon her.

And when they described recent episodes of illness, they tended, again very much more than other mothers, to describe the episode as the latest in a series, as something the child did get, or they said the child had a weakness, such as in the chest. Seventy-eight per cent of mothers with a persistently ill child ascribed a recent episode of illness to predisposition or history of such illness, compared to 16 per cent of other mothers.

> Ever since she was born she's had a bad chest. She's had a lot of coughs.
> Vomiting. He gets that. He's been in hospital because of him being sick so much.

She's allergic to some sorts of fruit, that's what must have brought on the rash.

He was crying and holding on to me, pulling his ear. It was hot – I felt it. I think it was the earache. Because he gets that. He's had it a lot over the last six or seven months.

So, not surprisingly, these mothers had particularly high levels of concern for their children's health, and about episodes of illness, and they felt they needed frequent consultation with the doctor to help them understand episodes and to try to protect the child both 'now' and for the future.

Support from social networks

It seemed possible that mothers with good social support would contact the doctor less quickly than others. They might consult friends and relatives first. Among the 135 mothers, 24 per cent said they did not have enough people to talk with about their child's health and welfare. So, we took those mothers (97) who said they had contacted the doctor in the last three months and grouped them according to whether or not they reported at least once contacting the doctor on the first day of the child's illness, and then set that against their satisfaction with their social support network.

This comparison showed that mothers who felt poorly supported were more likely than the rest to say they contacted the doctor on the first day of an illness: 71 per cent did once or more, compared to 45 per cent of the well-supported mothers. When this comparison was made, taking into account whether or not the mother had a persistently ill child, it was clear that first-day contact was strongly related to these two problems: persistent illness and having poor social support. In other words, these mothers felt they needed help quickly from the doctor because they had a child who caused them serious long-term worry *and* because they had few other people to turn to. For our sample, both these factors were commoner among classes III, IV and V than among classes I and II.

Constraints In Caring for Ill Children

Mothers have a busy life. They have to slot together all the many calls on their attention: child care, housework, shopping, paid work, preparing meals, social life, work commitments. Half the mothers (50 per cent) either had a second child or were pregnant, and for most of these child care was sometimes difficult because they were tired, or ill or worn down by children's behaviour. In addition, some mothers had been ill in other ways recently, and some fathers too. Some of the parents were under considerable strain because of chronic housing problems, inadequate income and unemployment.

Juggling commitments is often difficult enough even when children are well. Mothers' accounts show that if a child was ill they had to reassess their priorities, and in acute cases drop everything else to care for the child. During the last three months, most mothers told us about two, three or more occasions when they thought the child was ill or were concerned about the possibility of illness and so monitored the child more carefully. These conditions ranged from brief, trivial episodes to acute and worrying conditions that led to emergency calls on the health services.

The main problem in caring for ill children was that the mother was ill herself at the same time, either with the same condition, or often with pregnancy-related or childbirth-related illness.

> I had to send him to the minder anyway, even though he was ill (*with cough and cold*), because I just couldn't cope with him, straight after coming home with the baby.
>
> I had the flu as well, so I wasn't feeling very energetic.
>
> I haven't been able to pick her up, because I've been so weak with the pregnancy. (*Child with tonsillitis.*)
>
> I got it as well, and I was sick as well as her, the first night (*vomiting and diarrhoea*). My husband had to take time off to take her to the doctor.

Some of the mothers became more ill themselves, while caring for the ill child; their health problems were aggravated by tiredness and strain. Sleepless nights were common. In a few cases, the father was ill at the time of the child's illness, so the mother had two invalids to look after. Altogether, adult illness had been a problem during a child's illness for 33 per cent of the mothers.

The second major problem was related to paid work (15 per cent). Mothers had to stay away from work, and some mothers told unsympathetic employers the necessary lie: 'I rang them up and told them I had a cold'. Or else they were worried that the child was not getting consistent care if they shared the care with someone else. ('I was working full time, and Jennie (*the daily help*) was here, but I felt she needed constant care from just one adult.') Working mothers were worried about the child if they did arrange substitute care. ('She needed *me*, when she was ill.') Working parents coxed and boxed child care. ('I was worried, having been on (night) duty, about coping with him during the day. My husband was up with him on the night before.') Other kinds of work were difficult too:

> I couldn't really do anything, even make the dinner or pop out to do the shopping.

> I just had to sit and cuddle her all the time. I couldn't like go and do the washing up.

In some cases (11 per cent) the presence of a younger child in the household also made caring for the elder one more difficult. The ill child might be difficult to manage, because she was showing jealousy of the baby, or more jealousy than usual.

> She had a cold and she was being clinging and whining – more jealous of her sister, yesterday.

> There are times when she is deliberately boisterous for attention. When she wasn't feeling very well, she was very clinging to me, and she wouldn't stay at the playgroup. And I'm shorter tempered with her since I've had the baby.

> When he was waking at night with the teething, I had to take him into our bed, and it was waking the baby. He woke all of us. It was very tiring.

> When he was ill (*a cold*) I found it difficult to give him enough attention because I had the baby to look after.

These three sorts of problems – arising from adult ill health, from work commitments and from the care needs of a sibling were equally common in all classes. There was an additional set of problems which were commoner among households in classes III, IV and V, to do with poor housing (17 per cent) and poverty (12 per cent). As we showed in Chapter 3, getting help for ill children was difficult without a telephone or a car. But there were other problems too.

> I had to put her down in here (*in sitting room*) when she had the flu, to keep her away from the baby. So we were all upside down, trying to cope.

(*Child with diarrhoea, temperature and a virus.*) This house is cold. We had a problem keeping him warm.

(*Child with vomiting attack.*) We haven't got the facilities (*for washing and drying*). It's been difficult keeping up with all the extra washing, the bedding, the clothes.

(*Two children with coughs and temperature.*) Their room's so small. I had to have them in our room with me, and my husband slept on the sofa because he had to go to work next day. None of us got much sleep with them waking and the coughing.

(*Family living in homeless family hostel.*) He had the vomiting. And I had to bath him at 12 at night. It's a problem with all the other people living here.

We're finding it very difficult to manage at present. My husband's basic wage just about covers the basics. He's out a lot, doing overtime. If I'm not well, I still have to cope.

He needs a bit of fresh air when he's been ill, to set him up. But with the two of them, cramped up here (*3rd floor, no lift*) I can't get him out enough to run in the park.

Thus the household context within which mothers cared for ill children was perceived as important in affecting, and in some cases determining, how they cared for their ill children. Poor household resources were also perceived by mothers as adversely affecting children's health. Mothers explained that they could not afford to give the child good enough food to keep her in the best of health, and that they could not afford to buy safety equipment that they thought desirable. Housing conditions and poverty could lead to ill health:

You get some days they don't eat much, because of the weather, or whether they've had fresh air that day. If they've been in here all day they're not hungry. Then they won't eat a meal. (*2nd floor flat, no lift.*)

He gets a lot of colds in the winter. He gets run down in the winter. It's the central heating.

We can't keep a constant temperature in the house. We've had ice on the inside of the bedroom window, it's so cold. I have to light the gas (*cooker*) in the kitchen in the morning. It's not good for him.

We can't always keep him warm. He's continuously with us and it gets on your nerves a bit. Since Christmas we've all been sleeping on the front room floor to keep warm. His blankets keep getting damp and he comes in with us and it's a strain on our marriage. He won't even go in his own room. We all keep getting 'flu and colds. (*Mother says this child has weak valve in his chest and gets a lot of chest infections.*)

Mothers' accounts tell us that poor resources led to poor child health and they constrained child care. At each episode their children might be left less resistant to illness and their mothers were left less able to cope, because of increased ill health and the stress they lived under. Next time the child was ill the mother was less well able to look after her. Our analysis showed that where there were poor resources *and* a child with persistent illness, mothers were especially likely to report problems in caring for the ill child. In classes III, IV and V, most of those with a persistently ill child reported problems, compared to half of those whose children were not persistently ill (86 per cent against 54 per cent). There was no such difference for mothers in classes I and II.

Discussion

Mothers' accounts of their children's recent illnesses present a complex picture which suggests characteristics of their knowledge, patterns of care and pointers to explanation for class differences in care. Class differences overall in the reported incidence of acute illness and the number of days of illness in the study period (three months) were accounted for by the extra illnesses suffered by the persistently ill children, who came proportionately more from classes III, IV and V. Mothers of persistently ill children thought them vulnerable to illness and susceptible to recurrence of the persistent condition or to conditions associated with it. They consulted the doctor more often and at an early stage in episodes of illness. They tended to come from materially disadvantaged households, and had extra difficulties associated with poor housing and poverty in caring for ill children. No doubt their worries about the child and the constraints in caring interacted and compounded to make the worries and constraints yet more acute and burdensome.

Mothers managed most episodes of illness without professional help. As with other aspects of health care, they took responsibility for their children's welfare, and there was no tendency to rely on professionals to restore health. It seems likely that this self-reliance was a function of the skills and knowledge acquired over the first year or two of the child's life. Probably first-time mothers of younger children seek professional help more often. This point complements what many mothers said in connection with child health clinic services – they had needed frequent help at first but needed less now, for they had acquired knowledge and confidence.

Mothers' accounts also suggest that their beliefs about the seriousness of a condition related somewhat to the perceived site of the problem: the mouth, the chest, the stomach and bowels, and the skin. Thus mothers identified potentially serious symptoms such as high temperatures and diarrhoea and sometimes associated them with teething; because teething was considered a natural stage, and self-limiting, they did not usually consult a doctor. By contrast, conditions believed to be 'on' or potentially 'on' the chest were taken as serious, because the chest was perceived as vulnerable to infection. Anxiety about recurring respiratory infection in part explains our finding and that of Bax, Hart and Jenkins (1980): that mothers of children with persistent illness contacted the doctor more frequently than other mothers. It seemed that mothers expected the stomach and bowels to vary to some extent in their function for this age-range of children; at any rate they coped with loose stools and moderate diarrhoea unless there were other symptoms. Similarly, mothers seemed able to cope with skin disorders, once they had become familiar.

Mothers built up knowledge of what to do when a child was ill through experience and through discussion with other mothers. A few consulted books. Their knowledge of what a condition was to be called differed from that of professionals in most cases. Indeed (as shown in Chapter 9), a major reason for visiting the doctor was to get a diagnosis. Mothers wanted to know what label to put on it, for future reference, so that they would know what treatment was appropriate for what named condition, and just for peace of mind – to know if it was something to think of as serious (like bronchitis) or as trivial (like a cold). For those mothers with poor social support there were fewer opportunities to gain knowledge from discussion with friends and relatives.

There was almost no evidence of deference – not wanting to bother the doctor. Nor were mothers deterred from contacting the doctor because the service put up barriers to use. If they were worried they got professional help, though in some cases they turned to the hospital rather than the GP. But a third of mothers did find it difficult to know whether to contact a professional service. This can be seen as a natural process parents go through when a child develops symptoms, so in a sense this finding is not a matter for concern, for if they were worried they contacted a doctor.

Professionals to whom mothers turn for help will clearly be at an advantage in giving help if they recognize and respect mothers' knowledge about their children – the patterns of illness they have had, what symptoms now suggest cause for concern. Professionals should also be sensitive to the particular worries suffered by mothers whose children have long-term, chronic or recurrent conditions. These mothers are likely to seek help faster and more often than others. Finally, professionals should seek understanding of the circumstances in which mothers rear their children, and bear in mind that ill health, poverty and poor housing constrain mothers in caring for them. Professionals' ability to offer appropriate help to mothers will be enhanced or decreased according to their knowledge on these points. These topics will be taken up in the last two chapters of the book. But first the book will describe mothers' use of health services for their children.

Note to Chapter 8

1 Some mothers included accounts of behaviour problems or episodes of behavioural change; others did not. Because there may have been a pattern (e.g. by class) in who thought it appropriate to tell us about their children's behaviour, we have omitted data about behavioural episodes from the analysis, and included only physical conditions.

SECTION D

Using Health Services

Introduction

Chapters in this book so far have been about what mothers do to safeguard their children's health at home. The aim has been to consider what they thought important, what they knew about health care, what they did for their children, and what affected their child health care practices. These chapters have suggested some common themes about mothers' health care, and these themes in turn provide pointers to what mothers may value in health services.

First of all, mothers felt themselves to be in charge of their children's health. It was their job to safeguard their children, to keep them in good health and to restore them from illness to health. So while they turned to services for information, advice and treatment, this was on the understanding that they remained in charge. It seems likely, given this perspective, that mothers would want health service professionals to respect their views and to give full recognition to their responsibility for the child.

Secondly, mothers showed that they had high standards in health. Their account of an optimally healthy child was positive, rather than negative. They were interventionist and concerned to do well for their children. There was virtually no suggestion of apathy or hopelessness. So they would be likely to want health service staff to offer a commensurately high standard of service, one which aimed to keep the child in good health and was concerned for the individual child's welfare and progress.

Thirdly, our data show, not surprisingly, that the onset of child illness was often sudden and worrying. So mothers needed easily accessible services, which responded to their need for help, and which, again, recognized that if the customer asks for a service,

Introduction

there is usually a good reason for the request: the suddenness and severity of the condition and of the worry.

Fourthly, mothers' accounts indicate that child health care took place amid many other events, pressures and commitments. Mothers were busy people, juggling health care along with other responsibilities. So they would be grateful for services that were flexible in terms of hours and professionals who were flexible too, responding to mothers' need for help, both through surgery consultations and by home visiting.

Finally, there was evidence that mothers' knowledge on child health care did not always tally with what professionals might like them to know. Further, especially in respect of knowledge about illness, mothers indicated that they wanted to increase their knowledge, so they could care for their children well. So mothers needed opportunities to acquire knowledge, and for this they needed time to discuss illness, health and health care with people they trusted.

The above forms a long list. Some of the points made are self-evident, some perhaps less so. It is not, however, presented as a list of things the health services should do, but do not. Our data on mothers' perceptions of what constituted a good service and on whether they got it, suggest that health services were in general satisfactory to them. Nor is this list offered on the assumption that the customer's wishes and perceived needs ought to be met regardless of professional perspectives and of the constraints and circumstances within which professionals work. But one of the purposes of this book is to describe mothers' perspectives and to offer an account of what they think appropriate, and it is in this context that the data on use of health services are presented in the following chapters.

First, some notes on the health services available to the households in the study.

Health Services in the Study Area

The mothers in our sample lived in the catchment areas of two health centres, which covered about one-third of a district health authority's area.[1] The main *health services* used by mothers for their children are health centres, health visitors, general practitioners, hospitals, and to a small extent dentists. The information given here was the most up-to-date available for the field work period (1982). Most of it relates to the now defunct area health authorities.

It is difficult without conducting a detailed study to judge the quality of services. We thought the *health centres* in the study area were good, in a number of respects. First, according to the Medical Market Information's Directory of Health Centres (1982), which gives information sent in from health authorities, most districts have one or more health centres which offer a *wide range* of services, and others which offer just a few. Our district had six centres with this wide range, including the two chosen for this study. As far as mothers and children are concerned, the two health centres each offered routine child health clinic sessions, a creche, family planning, ante-natal care, a well-woman clinic, and one offered a drop-in advice service run by a psychologist, the other speech therapy. Each also had a dental service for children including under-fives and for women before and after childbirth. *Staffing* level is another possible indicator of quality. Most health centres have a group practice on the premises (three or more doctors; one of ours did, the other had two doctors). Most centres, like ours, have community nurses working from them (district nurses and health visitors). Another way of looking at quality is in terms of the furthest *distance* a family has to travel to a centre. Other studies have shown that distance from the centre affects use of it (Orr, 1980). In our area no one had more than a half-an-hour walk to get to the centre. It seems safe to assume that in our densely populated inner city area distances are less of a problem than in many other areas. Finally, on an anecdotal, personal level, *professionals* in child health told us they thought the services were relatively good and from our own exploration of possible study areas, we agreed with this verdict.

The importance of *health visitors* has long been recognized, but staffing levels have not met recommended targets. In inner London, where social needs point to the need for high numbers of health visitors, funded establishment levels are higher then elsewhere, and the Regional Health Authority (RHA) has recently set a target for the current ten years of a 22 per cent increase in health visitors. However, vacancy rates (judged against establishment levels) are higher than elsewhere (RHA unpublished data). Health visitors in inner London are likely to be unmarried, young and inexperienced compared to health visitors elsewhere. The annual rate of leaving or annual turnover rate at the time of this study was twice as high in inner London as in the home counties (27 per cent against 14 per cent) (Acheson Report, 1981).

In England and Wales generally four-fifths of health visitors work from GPs' practices (Dunnell and Dobbs, 1982) but in inner city areas, where there are fewer group practices, and where coverage of a mobile population is probably easier to achieve on an area basis, some district health authorities (DHAs) organize health visitors' work in 'patches' and they may work from health clinics and centres. In our area the ten health visitors who specialized in work with young families worked from the health centres, and covered a patch each, except for two who were attached to group practices. There were also four centre-based health visitors specializing in geriatric work.

Preventive child health services – advice for mothers for themselves and their under-fives, developmental checks and immunization – are provided at district health authority clinics and at GPs' well-baby clinics. Parents registered with a doctor offering this service may choose to use it, or may use the DHA clinic. Few of the doctors' practices in our DHA area (4 of 46) offered a well-baby clinic.

According to the Acheson Report (1981), inner London *General Practitioners* offer a poorer service on some criteria than those in outer London, or in England and Wales as a whole. Though there are enough doctors for the population judged by national standards, high proportions of them are elderly, few work in group practices and few have nurses working for them. Twice as many use deputizing services, rather than offer out-of-hours cover themselves. Informal evidence suggests that many of the doctors work in unattractive premises with poor facilities for patients (Acheson Report, 1981). High proportions work in single-handed practices (GLC, 1980). This picture was confirmed for the then area health authority from which our mothers chose their doctors: many doctors were aged 65 or more (23 per cent compared to 6 per cent for England); twice as many worked single-handed: just under one-third, compared to 16 per cent (RHA unpublished data). The proportion of doctors with nurses working for them was under half the national rate (Acheson Report, 1981).

In our area health authority area, as in the inner London AHAs generally, there is a high number of acute *hospital beds* for the population (GLC, 1980). People in the inner city also have access to the central specialist hospitals, such as Great Ormond Street (children), Moorfields (eye), Eastman's (dental). The inner London population is well served for hospital beds and for out-patient departments, although a high proportion of the people using the hospitals come from elsewhere. The main such groups are visitors, people from other areas referred for specialist services, and mobile people without their own GPs (GLC, 1980). The number of paediatric beds is high compared to other areas, but again the RHA notes that many are used by children from outside the area. The two hospitals most used by study parents for accidents and emergencies had no paediatric accident and emergency (A and E) department, but in one a paediatric specialist was on call. The hospitals were reasonably accessible; all study households had one within a mile and a half.

In general *what sort of a health service was it for mothers with young* children? This is a question to be addressed in the next two chapters of this book. But judging from the characteristics of the service mentioned above some initial comments can be made. Parents could get a service if they went to find it. Hospitals and doctors were available. Distances were not great, but if a mother wanted a service to come to her, things might not be so good. Many doctors did not offer 24-hour cover, and the deputizing service might be unreliable or impersonal and ineffective. If mothers wanted a reliable, caring person who knew them and was available at all times, then the services may not provide that. Single-handed doctors and elderly doctors might not be available to visit. If health visitor posts stayed vacant and a quarter of health visitors left their jobs each year, and if they were young and inexperienced, then mothers might not have the continuous support of a reliable, knowledgeable person who knew the family well.

From the *providers' point of view* it seems likely that working conditions in the health services in inner London will be constricting. For GPs, providing a responsive caring service will be hampered. Many doctors work from inconvenient cramped premises where it is hard to provide pleasant waiting rooms and good working space for receptionists and nurses. It is also difficult to get to know people on the list when the population is highly mobile. If health service professionals want to provide good preventive services, where they cover all children, diagnose and treat congenital conditions and help parents by teaching them about diet, dental care or accident prevention, then sufficient staff are needed, but may be lacking, to provide an accessible, flexible and acceptable service. If, as is commonly believed, some groups of parents are particularly reluctant to use preventive services, then helping them to see the virtue of doing so also requires expenditure of staff time. And in inner London there are high proportions of households thought to be low users of child preventive services: mobile families, families in classes IV and V, families with large numbers of children.

In the next two chapters mothers' use of curative and preventive services for their children is discussed.

Note to Section D

1 In order to maintain confidentiality, this account of the health services omits details that might identify the study area.

9

Contacts with Health Professionals

Introduction

Around the time of childbirth and in the first months of a child's life, health professionals intervene heavily in women's lives and women themselves seek help, especially for first babies. One way and another, women have a lot of contact with professionals during the year or two following the start of pregnancy. For mothers of older children, contacts with professionals may be less frequent, but are an accepted part of child rearing. Mothers are familiar with the varying purposes and practices of health service professionals: that they wish to carry out 'surveillance' of the children, will visit to check on children's welfare and may suggest certain child-care practices, as well as that they are there to respond to requests for help. Mothers in this study viewed health services as useful and important sources of advice, information and treatment. They felt the services were there for them to use – and they did use them when they were worried about their children's health.

This chapter is about mothers' use of health services for their children. It considers their opinions on GPs and health visitors, their access to help from GPs and hospitals, and their recent experiences of meetings with GPs, health visitors and hospital staff. Mothers' views and experiences are considered in the light of what has been learned from their health care of their children at home about their perspectives on health services. They will appreciate services which respect their wishes and value their

GPs and Health Visitors

The GPs

All the 135 mothers said they had registered their children with a doctor or with a practice, in most cases the one they went to themselves (97 per cent). Between them they were registered with 59 doctors. According to the mothers, most of the children (84 per cent) were registered with a particular GP, the rest with a practice. The doctors or practices each had on average 2.3 of the study children on their lists (range 1 to 12). Forty-five of the doctors had only one or two of the children.

In important respects, these doctors were not typical of those in the health district in general and some worked outside the district. Most (63 per cent) of the district's doctors work in ones or twos and nearly a quarter are aged 65 or more. However according to the mothers, their doctors worked mainly in groups of three or more (65 per cent) and only 6 per cent of them were over 65. Jefferys and Sachs' (1983) findings suggest a reason for this marked difference. They found that people aged 15–34 (the age-range of 81 per cent of our sample) tended to go to group practices. Probably they prefer the range and greater flexibility of the service offered. Possibly also older doctors are less likely than younger to have made the transition to working in group practices. Some of the mothers had chosen group practices partly because these tended to offer a variety of services and some had a doctor who specialized in paediatric work.

Asked what they liked or disliked about the doctor's practice, most mothers commented on the arrangements for seeing the doctor – making an appointment, or waiting your turn (see Table 9). The quality of staff – doctors, receptionists, and nurses was important. Staff should be kindly, concerned and competent. Mothers appreciated being made welcome, having a reasonable place to wait and not having to wait too long. It was important for some mothers that the practice offered a range of

Table 9.1 *Proportions of mothers who mentioned various features of the GP's practice as important*

Features mentioned	Type of comment Favourable	Adverse	Proportion who mentioned this feature
Arranging to see doctor	40	23	63
Quality of staff	34	20	54
Pleasant place	23	25	48
Waiting times	14	26	40
Variety of services	36	1	37
Welcoming	30	6	36
Service to children	21	5	26

No. of mothers = 126.

services under one roof, such as ante-natal care, a child health clinic, family planning. And a few mothers stressed that they valued an expert service for children. Sizeable minorities of the mothers thought the practice was poor as regards arranging to see the doctor, quality of staff, physical conditions and waiting times. And like other studies, this one found that twice as many mothers in classes I and II as of other mothers were critical about physical conditions (37 per cent against 17 per cent) and waiting times (39 per cent against 17 per cent). However, these were comments at a general level, and it may be that the class difference reflects a willingness by some mothers to generalize, or to set the actual service against an ideal. For the most recent visit to the doctor there were no class differences in waiting times or complaints about them.

Health visitors

According to the mothers, health visitors offered a widely varying service. For a start, though all the mothers had a GP for their children, only 72 per cent considered they had a health visitor. That is, an important minority said there was no health visitor who was 'theirs'. Possibly the health visitors had these mothers on their lists and thought they had made sure the mother knew who they were and how to contact them, but if so, this perception did not match the mothers'. It seems that within this age-range of children, health visitors concentrated their resources on families they thought especially needed help. This is in line with suggested practice by the Health Visitors' Association (1981). While almost all the mothers in classes IV and V said they had a health visitor (89 per cent), lower proportions of mothers in the other class groups said so (57 per cent to 77 per cent). It also seems that health visitors had visited these mothers at home more recently. Though only 30 per cent of all the mothers said they had been visited at home in the last three months, 54 per cent of those in classes IV and V had had a visit, compared to a quarter of the other mothers.

The service also varied in terms of continuity. Nearly a third of the mothers had had the same health visitor since their child was born, but most of the rest had had two or more, although five mothers said they had never had a health visitor as far as they knew. One reason why mothers change their health visitor is if they move house – and this accounted for a third of the 96 changes. But according to the mothers most of the changes took place because the health visitor left the job or was transferred to another post or health centre. (A member of the nursing management staff also pointed to high rates of maternity leave as an important factor at the time of the study.)

So some mothers had known their present health visitor for much longer than others had. Forty-two per cent had known her for over 18 months, including 29 per cent who had had the same health visitor for all their child's lifetime. At the other end of the scale, 10 per cent had known her for less than six months and 28 per cent had no health visitor.

What is the health visitor's job?
Both the GP and the health visitor are well established figures in mothers' lives, but while in general the GP responds to requests for help, the health visitor *proffers* a service; indeed she asks to come in and talk with you, just because you have a young child. Almost all the mothers (92 per cent) thought one of her roles was to help them with what they themselves identified as problems. The health visitor should be an expert in child care and development who could be called upon to discuss and help with major and minor problems. The mothers saw the health visitor as being there for their benefit. Some mothers (43 per cent) also thought

the health visitor's job was to be a generally supportive person, whom they could rely on for help, both for specific problems and for reassurance, as a friendly member of staff within the health service. ('She's somebody who's there if you're worried about something.')

A second side of the health visitor's job was identified by 61 per cent of mothers: it was to inspect, and to make sure the children were well cared for. This function seemed to be readily accepted by most of the mothers who mentioned it.

> She wouldn't like it, but I think she's there to check up on me. It's a good thing for the sake of the children. It doesn't bother me, but that's basically it. That's part of the job. It's like being a social worker – they check to see the home's OK.

The implication was that the health services had a right to monitor parental care and to intervene if they saw the need. But a few mothers (15 per cent) described this function in ways that suggested an unwelcome intrusion. The health visitor's job was to check up on you, spy on you, look to see if you'd slipped up, or to catch you out.

> She should be concerned with the children. She should be helpful about problems – like housing. But they're nosy, interfering.

> They come round to inspect, check up on you. They're always looking round to see what the place is like. I didn't like the way she looked about – to see if she could see anything wrong.

A few mothers (10 per cent) also saw the health visitor as someone who was there to instruct mothers, whether they liked it or not, in what she saw as good child care.

The third main kind of job identified by mothers was that of encouraging or helping families in their use of services – both the health service and other services. The health visitor was seen as a liaison person, who reminded you about health centre appointments and could ease the way towards getting pre-school care for a child, or could help negotiations with the housing department.

Mothers differed according to their class background in their views on the health visitor's job. Mothers in classes I and II were more likely than others to think of the health visitor as helping them with problems they identified (78 per cent against 62 per cent), and very much more likely to see her as offering support

(48 per cent against 21 per cent). Mothers in classes IV and V were more likely than the rest to see the health visitor as an investigator – 65 per cent of them thought the job was to make sure children were well cared for, compared to 42 per cent of the other mothers. And, compared to the other mothers, rather more of those in classes III, IV and V talked about the health visitor as an unwelcome teacher, or as someone who checked up on mothers (20 per cent compared to 13 per cent; not statistically significant). It seems very likely that this difference in perception derives from mothers' different circumstances and different experiences of health visitors. Well-to-do mothers in pleasant homes may feel able to raise their children well. If health visitors are critical of them, the mothers may feel confident enough about their child-rearing capabilities to shrug off criticism. Nor is it so likely that they or their friends will have seen the sharper edge of the health visitor's job. In addition, some of these mothers had as much child-care book learning as the health visitor, if not more. So the meetings between them were probably seen as between equals, and mothers might direct discussion to what they wanted to discuss, rather than follow the health visitor's lead. Mothers in classes IV and V were more vulnerable to the inspecting side of the health visitor. Some had poor housing for rearing children, many were hard pressed financially. Many were younger than the health visitors, less well educated and perhaps less able to stand up for themselves. The possibility of intervention in family life was real to some mothers. Mothers' accounts of recent contact with health visitors indicated that they had intervened in some cases on housing and pre-school care, and on more personal family problems. Some of this intervention was welcome, some not, but it probably influenced mothers' perceptions of the health visitor's job.

However this may be, mothers' different perceptions of the health visitor's job throw into relief the difficulties of providing a good, acceptable service. Her job is interventionist, whether she is offering support or inspecting. How is she to provide general support and friendly discussion of mothers' problems if she is also acting as an inspector, or thinks she must try to change mothers' behaviour? Some parents whom health visitors think are especially in need of help may reject unwelcome kinds of intervention. As noted above, 15 per cent of mothers opposed the interventionist principle of health visiting.

Table 9.2 *Proportion of mothers who mentioned qualities of their GP and health visitor*

	GP[a]			HV[b]		
	Positive comment	Negative comment	Total	Positive comment	Negative comment	Total
Respects mother's views	47	12	59	40	6	46
Thorough/follows up request	50	6	56	33	6	39
Nice	42	13	55	61	3	64
Is a 'family doctor'/ takes personal interest	37	8	45	29	1	30
Good with children	40	4	44	9	1	10
Knowledgeable	36	5	41	21	8	29
Willing to inform	30	9	39	44	3	47
Knowledgeable about children	15	1	16	22	4	26
Willing to do visit at home	16	3	19	24	7	31

[a] Number of mothers = 114. [b] Number of mothers = 94.
Note: 114 mothers were registered with a particular GP and 94 had a health visitor.

'Good' doctors and 'good' health visitors

Three-quarters of the GPs and health visitors were described as 'good' by the mothers, without reservation. Their descriptions of good and bad qualities in these health professionals suggest what mothers valued (see Table 9.2).

Their values for each professional were somewhat similar. Personal qualities and thoroughness in the job were important for both doctor and health visitor. Willingness to give information and to respect mothers' views were mentioned by many mothers. It is notable that mothers were concerned that doctors, but not health visitors, should be good with children. A mother often has to let the doctor handle her child, so behaviour acceptable to the child is important. It is also notable that there were more adverse ratings of doctors than of health visitors; few health visitors got any adverse comments and then usually only one; whereas a few doctors came in for several criticisms, notably that they were not nice, friendly people and that they did not respect the mothers' views.

There were no class differences in all this except that for both GPs and health visitors mothers in classes I and II were much more likely than other mothers to emphasize that a doctor should be knowledgeable, and mothers in classes III, IV and V were more likely to say a doctor should be willing to inform and a health visitor to respect their views. Possibly this is a matter of wording – you do not know if someone is knowledgeable unless he tells you something – but it does tie in with other findings. For instance, there was a very clear class trend in proportions of mothers who praised a doctor or practice that offered a child-oriented service – from 53 per cent in class I to 12 per cent in classes IV and V. These mothers said they valued having specialist knowledge available. However, as we shall see, accounts of recent visits to the doctor show that many mothers voiced concern that the doctor should behave sensitively to the child. The emphasis by some groups of mothers on wanting respect for their opinions may reflect the fear or experience of being disrespected and this may be commoner among those who in class terms are distant from professionals. As has been noted, some mothers in classes III, IV and V thought the health visitor's job was partly to inspect, and their accounts of recent visits show they thought this function was in evidence.

All in all, 49 per cent of the mothers thought they had either a good doctor or a good health visitor, and 38 per cent thought both were good. At the other extreme, 13 per cent felt neither were good or, more commonly, they had a poor doctor and no health visitor. So nearly two-fifths had two trusted professionals to turn to, half had one and a few no one. There were no differences by class, education or the child's age on this point.

Establishing friendly relations is probably important if mothers are to trust their health professionals, but perhaps the personal relationship matters even more with a health visitor than with a doctor, since she is perceived by mothers to offer a response to their needs. Such a relationship allows mothers to raise and discuss in detail the many problems and decisions they face in child care, which are often complex and affect several people's welfare, and so require careful consideration and sensitive management. Continuity did seem to be important in affecting mothers' rating of the health visitor: 90 per cent of those who had

had the same health visitor for all the child's life thought she was good, compared to 65 per cent who had known her for shorter periods.

There was no relationship between mothers' rating of the doctor and how long they had known the doctor. Possibly people do not expect to get on well personally with doctors. However, when it came to assessing the recent visit to the doctor, it was mothers who saw the child's own doctor who thought the visit was satisfactory.

Access to Professional Help

Distance and transport

Most of the mothers (81 per cent) lived within a fifteen minute journey of their GP and most walked to the surgery (71 per cent). Few mothers, mostly in classes I and II, had access to a car during the week (24 per cent) and the minority who went to the doctor's by car (19 per cent) were almost all mothers in classes I and II. All the mothers had a health centre within a half hour's walk and all were able to get to a hospital within half an hour, mostly more quickly if need be. For emergency trips to the hospital – for accidents and sudden onset illness – mothers had gone by car (their own or a friend's) or by taxi and none complained of difficulties in getting to hospital. So for getting help for children, parents were probably fairly well placed, at least in comparison with people living in a small town or country district. But some mothers had difficulties getting their child to the doctor. Of the 71 who had taken her in the last three months, 20 per cent said their journey was difficult. This was because the weather was bad, or because managing two children, at least one of whom was ill, was difficult. Mothers had to weigh the advantages of talking with a doctor against the disadvantage, as they saw it, of perhaps aggravating the illness by taking the child out.

Arranging a meeting

On the whole mothers turned to GPs or hospital doctors rather than to health visitors for professional help with ill children, but arranging to see a doctor at the surgery was not always straightforward. Some doctors had appointment systems and 27 per cent referred to these, with about half liking and half disliking them. However, of those who commented on a first-come-first-served system (31 per cent), four-fifths approved of it; on balance the advantage of being seen, even after a long wait, outweighed the advantage of making an appointment and of being seen, usually more quickly, for mothers had found they could not always get an appointment when they needed it. As noted in Chapter 3, arranging to see a health professional was easier if mothers had access to both a telephone and car. For those without day-time access to either, the disadvantages of having to go to the surgery to make an appointment (leaving a sick child at home) and then go again with the child, inclined them to favour the no appointments system.

Waiting to see the doctor was another aspect of the doctor's practice that some mothers commented on; 14 per cent thought waiting times in general were reasonable but 26 per cent thought they were not. Mothers' accounts of their most recent visit show that over half (55 per cent) thought they had waited for less than 15 minutes, 26 per cent for up to half an hour and 19 per cent for longer periods – up to two hours in a few cases. There were no class differences in waiting times or satisfaction with them on that occasion.

The mothers' stories of the most recent visit to the doctor also showed that many found difficulties in their way before they managed to see the doctor. In some cases this was because surgery hours did not fit in well with the mothers' daily routines and job. Or if there was an appointment system, they could not get an appointment for that day. Mothers without a telephone talked of the problems of making an appointment. Some said they had to wait a long time, sometimes in what they described as unpleasant, cramped and crowded conditions. Nine mothers found their route to the doctor blocked by the receptionist, who tried to discourage them from seeing the doctor. Altogether 31 per cent of the mothers mentioned one or more of these problems, and this was commoner among mothers in classes III, IV and V where nearly half (44 per cent) reported problems, compared to 15 per cent of other mothers.

Few mothers (15 per cent) said they had turned to a health visitor for help with illness in the last three months. This may be commoner among mothers of younger children. In the study area, one of the health centres runs a popular walk-in service staffed by health visitors to advise mothers with health problems and to refer them on to the doctor if either mother or health visitor thinks that useful. However, 16 per cent of mothers said they had asked health visitors for help of various other kinds in the last three months. Either they sought help at the clinic, or they asked for a health visitor to visit them at home – and all these requests for a visit had been met. Mothers asked for discussion about the child's behaviour – eating and sleeping problems, and about housing, financial and relationship difficulties.

Getting a home visit

Apart from those few mothers who had actively sought out help from the health visitor, it seemed most mothers did not initiate contact with the health visitor. Only 20 per cent of recent visits from the health visitor were requested by the mother. Mothers waited to be visited, perhaps because when the baby was first born they had received unsolicited visits. But 38 per cent commented that they rarely saw a health visitor, and 13 per cent said they wished they did, because they could do with advice or discussion.

However, mothers did sometimes ask for visits from the GP. Of the 135 mothers, most (61 per cent) had at some time asked for a visit for the study child. If we take the most recent of these requests (the most recent for each mother), for 80 per cent of them the doctor came. The few cases (16) where the doctor did not come suggest a mismatch between mothers' and doctors' perceptions about who should decide that a child needs a home visit. All the requests but one were made in the day-time or during evening surgery. Three receptionists answered the phone and suggested that the mothers come to the surgery. The rest of the mothers spoke to the doctor and she or he assessed the situation and asked the mother to bring the child to the surgery if she was worried. Almost all the mothers were dissatisfied with this – after all they had asked for a visit because they thought the child too ill to be taken out, because the weather was bad, because they would have had to take their young baby too, or because they thought the child might be infectious. So these were cases where the mother's view was overridden by the GP or the receptionist. Twelve of these mothers followed the doctor's advice and took the child to the surgery. It seems reasonable that the doctor (but perhaps not the receptionist) should share with the parents the decision about whether a home visit is necessary. But the residue of dissatisfaction in the mothers who were not visited might deter them in future from asking and so lead to a trip to the hospital or to delayed consultation for a seriously ill child.

Getting help at the hospital

These inner city mothers had an extra source of help for their children: the hospital. Apart from visits for specialist advice – to both local and slightly more distant hospitals, the mothers (and fathers) used the hospital in two main circumstances: for sudden onset illness and for accidents.

If we take the most recent visit to a hospital in the last twelve months, then 62 children went to an out-patient or to an accident and emergency department. Sixteen of these visits were for sudden or suddenly worsening illness. While there were no class differences in the numbers taken to specialist departments, or for accidents, there was a class difference on this. Fourteen of the 16 children came from classes III, IV and V.

So it seems that a small proportion of the mothers (12 per cent) used the hospital for conditions about which others might perhaps have consulted the GP. The number of cases is small, but some comments can be made. Some of the 16 mothers had seen their GP that day and had a letter to take to the hospital; others had seen their GP, felt reassured and then found that the illness got much worse in the evening. Most of these hospital visits took place late in the evening, or at weekends, and it is notable that mothers registered with single- or double-handed practices were more likely than mothers at group practices to take their child along to the hospital. The small number of mothers in the sample with no telephone were also highly represented among these 16 mothers. One-fifth of them just took their child along compared to one-tenth of those with a telephone. All of this suggests reasons why the mothers took their children. It is known that people do not like the deputizing services used by GPs out of surgery hours, and these are more likely to be used by doctors who work alone or in pairs (Acheson Report, 1981, para. 3.59). Dislike of deputizing services, coupled with the problem of making contact if mothers have no telephone, probably accounts for some of the visits.

The other reason for turning to the hospital was for accidents. We asked mothers to tell us the story of the most recent accident to the child in the last three months. Most of these 66 accidents were minor and the mother dealt with it herself, or with help from fathers, friends and relatives. But in 13 cases she sought professional help. In most of these cases the child had, she thought, sustained an injury to some part of the head and she thought there might be serious injury. It is notable that for ten of these 13 accidents mothers turned not to the GP but to the hospital. This seemed to be because first, whatever help was needed, the hospital's resources would be able to cope – with X-rays, in-patient treatment, specialist diagnosis; and secondly, because the parents could be sure the child would be seen, even if it took some time. There was no restriction at the hospital to certain hours.

Visits to and from Professionals

A visit to the doctor

We asked mothers to tell us about the most recent visit to the doctor for their children in the last three months. As with the information on symptoms, we asked for the story of the visit and prompted to cover the topics we thought important too. Of the 135 children 71 (53 per cent), equally by class, had been taken to the doctor during this period, all but two by their mother. In general, the mothers were happy with the visit and their accounts suggest a competent, caring and reasonably flexible service. But there were some drawbacks and some mothers were less satisfied than others.

What did mothers go *about*? Virtually all the visits were about medical conditions and worries. The biggest single problem was respiratory conditions (32 per cent), followed by skin conditions (16 per cent). The rest of the mothers took their children because they were 'ill', distressed or had a high temperature (25 per cent) or had a suspected infectious disease or other illness (14 per cent). Only 3 mothers (4 per cent) took their children for behaviour problems. The remaining 9 per cent of visits were for other, mixed reasons.

What did mothers go *for*? They went for a variety of purposes, some for more than one purpose. Some went simply to get a prescription (mostly for coughs) or for a repeat of an earlier prescription. Some went specifically for the doctors' technical expertise, to ask him to examine the child's chest, or look down his ears. Or they went to get a diagnosis – to have a name put on the condition – to find out that it was nothing worse than a cough and cold, or that it *was* the measles. ('Once I'd taken her and found out what it was, and that it would clear up, it eased my mind.') But of course many mothers went to discuss the child's condition – what was the appropriate treatment, or how long would the condition last. Some mothers wanted reassurance, and the chance to talk to a sympathetic expert.

Most mothers were happy with the outcome as regards getting a prescription, an examination of the child or a diagnosis. But there was more dissatisfaction among those who wanted to discuss the child's condition. Mothers' explanation for this was not that the doctors, in the main, seemed uncaring, but that they gave the impression of being in a hurry.

> We was in there about two minutes. He listened to his chest – through his clothes. He looked down his throat. He just said – he prescribed the same medicine he always prescribes. He didn't say anything at all. I don't think he really likes giving prescriptions. I didn't say anything to him. He makes you feel he doesn't want to see you. Really rushed.

This impression is clearly documented in the mothers' assessment of the doctor's behaviour during the consultation. Few of the mothers thought their doctor was cold or unfriendly or unhelpful or unsympathetic (fewer than 15 per cent for each behaviour), but over a third (36 per cent) thought she or he seemed to be in a hurry. The effect of this was to make some mothers (27 per cent) feel that they did not have enough time to discuss the problem. ('I didn't feel he had enough time for me, or for my child. He just didn't give us time to talk about it.') Some mothers (22 per cent) were left with the feeling that the doctor did not respect their views.

The other main drawback to the consultation was the doctor's behaviour with the child. Most mothers' accounts of the consultation included a description of how the child felt and how she reacted to the doctor's behaviour. Clearly mothers felt for their child, who was ill or distressed anyway and liable to be further upset if treated insensitively. So mothers made a point of describing how the doctor behaved with the child. Mostly this was praise. For instance:

He said 'hello'. We said 'hello'. He greets you friendly. Knows your name immediately. I described Janice's cold and the cough. She was sitting on my knee. And he made jokes and showed her pens and got her interested and then he listened to her chest.

But a substantial minority of mothers (17 per cent) thought the doctor's behaviour was insensitive and that the examination of the child was poor (20 per cent) – mainly again because the doctor was too sudden, or rough, or did not talk to the child.

He said to me 'What's wrong?' I said, 'She's got a cough'. He said, 'Let me examine her'. He went to examine her straightaway. Never said hello to the child. She went hysterical. He was getting annoyed, I was getting annoyed, because she'd never cried before with my own doctor. I was fuming, really upset, because I didn't like the way he treated her at all.

Taking the consultation as a whole, half the mothers (56 per cent) were completely satisfied, 21 per cent had some reservations and 24 per cent were dissatisfied. Here are two satisfied customers:

I was most impressed. She was most relaxed. She took the time, even though it was right at the end of the surgery. And she showed sensitivity to the child. She was very thorough.

He's very good. I felt reassured. I have confidence in him because he tells me what's happening. He'll tell the truth and not pretend.

And a dissatisfied one:

It was very upsetting. He made me feel I was some irresponsible mother – as if I had caused it – it seems he hasn't got time for anyone. He just wants to get you in and get you out. He said 'I'll look in her ears' – he said, 'Will you *please* hold her still'. He near enough had a go at me – he said 'What have you been giving her'?

Some of the worst encounters were with unfamiliar doctors. The child's own doctor was not on duty, or the child was registered with the practice not with a particular doctor.

He was plain off-hand and quite rude. He was prepared to prescribe something without even looking at him. I felt he wasn't really doing his job ... He didn't try to make it any easier for Peter – useless, hopeless.

Familiarity seems to be important – most mothers were satisfied with the consultation if they saw the child's own doctor (64 per cent) whereas only 38 per cent of those who saw another doctor were satisfied.

Mothers from different class groups were equally satisfied and dissatisfied with the various aspects of the consultation described here, and were equally satisfied overall. The only class difference was a tendency for the mothers in classes IV and V to be less critical of the doctor's manner than the rest (but the numbers are small).

A visit from the health visitor

Most mothers had some contact with health visitors and 60 per cent said they had spoken with a health visitor in the last three months, at the clinic or at home. Since clinic contacts are very varied in character and in duration, we asked mothers instead to tell us the story of the most recent visit at home in the last three months. There were 40 of these, and, as noted above, mothers in classes IV and V were more likely than other mothers to have been visited, no doubt because they were perceived to be in need of a visit. Possibly too health visitors singled out for visits mothers thought to be poorly supported, for they had visited rather more of those mothers who told us they had insufficient people to talk with about their child (42 per cent had had a visit compared to 25 per cent of the rest).

According to the mothers, most of the visits (80 per cent) were on the health visitor's initiative and most were made without an appointment. Usually, mothers welcomed the visit.

> It was a surprise to see her. (*Family had just moved house.*) But it was nice to know someone cares and takes an interest in you.
>
> It was nice to have someone to talk to.
>
> I enjoyed it.

We cannot of course say what the health visitor saw as the purpose of the visit, but mothers seemed to have a clear idea about it. Some visits (at least ten) were specifically to see the new baby.

> I came home from hospital on the Friday and she called round on the Monday but I was out and she came back on the Tuesday. And she asked me generally how I was and looked at the baby – her belly button and her head and eyes. And I told her her motions were a bit

hard and she said give her plenty of fluid and not to worry. I was a bit worried. She said only to worry if she was sick and she hasn't been.

We chatted about the birth. I had no problems or questions. We just chatted and she looked at the baby and asked how she was. I gave her a cup of tea. It was like a social visit. It was very nice.

In at least seven visits discussion centred on a family health problem. Some of the health visitors were following up a concern about a member of the family.

She just called round. I made her a cup of coffee. She mainly played with Paul for about an hour. He read books to her and she played cars with him. He was telling her the Argos catalogue, the toys in it ... It was fine. It was company for the afternoon. She came mainly for him, because she couldn't get a word out of him at the clinic the Wednesday before. So she more or less came to make sure he was alright. She might have thought, deep down, that he was feeling a bit pushed out because of the baby – but she didn't say anything – it's just what I think.

She came because I'd been to the clinic because I was bleeding (*in early pregnancy*). So she came. It was a follow-up. She asked how I was. She didn't stay long. We just chatted about it. And she asked how he was. It was very nice that she came. I was very happy to talk about what had been happening to me.

Or the mother asked for a visit:

I went to talk to her about – we're planning to have another baby. And I had a lot of difficulty having him and I still feel a lot of it was to do with the drugs I was given ... And she said she'd come round because she didn't have enough time at the clinic. And she came and she stayed for a couple of hours and we talked it through and she gave me a book of her own to read, about induced labour. She was very good. She was very caring all round.

In ten cases, all with mothers in classes IIIb, IV and V, the mothers said the main topic of conversation was housing, day care, family relationships or money. In some cases health visitors offered not just advice but practical help – with finding a day-care place, help with housing problems. They gave mothers useful telephone numbers and discussed tactics for solving problems. In one case the health visitor gave particularly useful practical help.

She came in, she told me the doctor had told her about the accident (to child's father). She was very kind. Very helpful. I was in terrible tension. She took me up to the Social Services Department in her car to tell them about it. I couldn't have managed alone – I was on my own with the children. I was very grateful. I really needed some help. She was marvellous.

These visits were very different in character from visits to the doctor's surgery, which were seen as being for one or more specific purpose; discussion was limited to the child's physical condition. During the visit from the health visitor mothers were on their own home ground. The health visitor was the mother's guest – to be given a cup of tea and made welcome. Unless the health visitor showed signs of being in a hurry or the mother was busy herself, it seems there was a relatively relaxed atmosphere in which many topics could be raised by either side and in which health care of the child was considered in its social context. Mothers were well aware that the health visitor was doing a job, which included checking up on child care and child development, but in general they accepted that this was for the benefit of the children. And most of the health visitors were described as pleasant, friendly and genuinely concerned for both adults and children. However, there were differences by class in mothers' satisfaction with the visit. Most mothers (67 per cent) found the visit helpful, or were happy with what took place, although 18 per cent thought the visit was rushed, but mothers in classes IV and V were much less likely than the rest to be satisfied. What they disliked was made clear in their ratings of the health visitor's manner. Some of them saw her as unfriendly, unhelpful, unsympathetic and not concerned for them.

She just came in. She just walked in. She asked how Charlie was keeping and how I was. I didn't mind. But she was criticizing me. She didn't bother to come for two months and then she came without an appointment. She wasn't helpful. Impertinent.

Dissatisfaction with the health visitor's visit was also linked to having a persistently ill child, though less strongly than to class. Perhaps mothers were unable to get effective help for these children and this accounts for some of their dissatisfaction.

Judging from these accounts by mothers of home visits by health visitors, it seems that while for many mothers the health visitor was seen as helpful and friendly, this was less likely for socially disadvantaged mothers – many of whom might be in great need of help. If they did need help, their poor relationship with the health visitor might mean they had one less person to turn to.

A visit to the hospital

Sixty-two children were taken to hospital once or more in the last twelve months, as out-patients, mostly to the two nearest hospitals to the study area. Thirty-six went to the accident and emergency department and 26 to specialist out-patient departments. Most of the visits were for emergencies – for accidents (39 per cent of cases) or for sudden, or suddenly worsening illness (23 per cent). These emergency visits were made without an appointment, though in a few cases the GP had suggested the visit. Most of the rest of the visits were by appointment and were for specialist diagnosis and check-up. As noted earlier mothers in classes III, IV and V were especially likely to take their children for sudden onset illness. But there was no class difference in the proportions of children taken for accidents, or for specialist consultations.

Mothers of persistently ill children were especially likely to seek help from the hospital for their children. In particular they took their children when there was a recurrence, or suspected recurrence of the condition that caused long-term concern. The story told by Jean's mother (below) shows why she turned to the hospital for help. Her worry about a suspected recurrence of bronchitis, as well as other factors led her to seek help there immediately, rather than wait to see the doctor.

Almost all the emergency visits were to hospitals with a *general* (not a children's) accident and emergency department. This made the visit particularly difficult for mothers and fathers with an ill or hurt child. They had to wait in a bleak crowded room or corridor (with drunks waltzing around, said one mother), with no facilities for keeping children amused or quiet. Parents felt their child should be given priority over adults because they were in such distress. Some felt that nurses and doctors were inexpert – 'very young', 'you could tell he was newly qualified' – and that they lacked skills in caring for children or in talking with parents of distressed children. However, half of those who went without an appointment were satisfied overall with the visit mainly because in the end they got a good medical service, or because they did not have to wait too long.

Satisfaction with the visit was much more likely if mothers had an appointment. Virtually all those with an appointment were satisfied (91 per cent), compared to 53 per cent of those who just went along, irrespective of class. The more detailed findings on mothers' satisfaction suggest why this is so. Most mothers were satisfied with the examination of the child (82 per cent), most thought the doctor respected their views (83 per cent) and most thought they had enough time to discuss the problem (76 per cent). For the first two there was no difference in mothers' satisfaction whether they went with an appointment or not, but those who went without an appointment were likely to feel they had insufficient time to discuss the problem. Mothers found a busy, sometimes hectic scene, with tired, harassed staff, who rushed them through. Doctors seen by appointment had more time to give.

> He examined her very nicely. I was very impressed by his personality, with his receptive abilities. He listened, he took notice of what I said. Included us all, me, my husband and Michelle – he talked to her. She wasn't just an object.
>
> The doctor was very good. He let me tell him what I thought was wrong with her. Then he explained everything.
>
> I was more than pleased with the doctor. He'll spend as much time as you need.
>
> She spent some time talking to Emma and establishing a relationship with her.

A further point here emerged from mothers' stories about the trip to the hospital. A third of those with no appointment (compared to one of those with one) said that during the visit a nurse or doctor called in question their behaviour as a parent: why had they brought the child, why had they not brought her earlier, why had they let the accident happen; or the parents' advice on how to manage the distressed child was rejected. The professionals' behaviour may have been a reaction to stressful working conditions, or a response to seeing distressed children. Parents saw this criticism as unjustified, when they had done their best by getting the child to hospital.

> (*Child with vomiting and temperature at 10 months.*) He said 'Why did you bring her here? There's nothing wrong with her.' I said the child has a temperature. He said, what do you want me to do about it?

He was a bit cheeky. He wasn't very nice. He said why didn't you call in your own doctor? It's not the right thing to jump in a taxi and bring her here – it's an emergency department, for accidents. You can't just come to the hospital with no letter. You should have called your own doctor in. And your own doctor could have given you a letter. You don't just come to casualty. I was really angry. I said if your child was sick – with a temperature, what would you do?

She said it was my fault because I didn't have her immunized. (*Child with whooping cough.*)

She just examined his stomach very quickly that was all, not very thorough. She didn't give us time to talk, she just told us off, I think because I've read you should be careful with babies when they get diarrhoea not to let them get dehydrated. It was very upsetting, she was quite rude ... She asked us horrible questions which didn't relate to what was wrong. She asked us if we had any more children and we said no and she said we were overreacting.

They kept asking me how I came to let her take the pills. At first I was so upset, I thought they were blaming me. Afterwards I knew they had to find out how she took them.

To understand why mothers took their children to hospital it is important to know something of the background of the visit. This next mother's account of her daughter Jean's recent illness and of her circumstances provide explanations of her actions. Three months previously the family returned from Scotland. They were homeless. The father was unemployed and chronically sick. The family was housed by the council in one room in a hostel. They were still registered with the doctor two miles away near their previous dwelling, but had a 'temporary' arrangement with a doctor near the hostel. The mother thought the doctor was good, but complained (like other mothers using the practice) that you had to wait 'hours' to see him. The family was sharing all amenities with other families in the hostel, they had no car, but the use of the hostel phone. Soon after they moved in:

She wouldn't eat. It lasted a week. And she wouldn't sleep. I was worried. She was crying a lot. She was fretting for her gran. I thought she'd die. I called the health visitor. She was only drinking milk. The health visitor said if she's hungry she'll eat. I thought there must be something wrong with her after two days. I took her to the doctor after two days. He said lots of children go through this. In fact when the health visitor came up, two days later, she ate a whole loaf of bread in front of her and made me out a liar. When my brother came to see us, she went (*as if*) she wanted to go with him. She's still not sleeping. Since we came back (*from Scotland*) it's been going on. I've found her all strange – she's not sleeping in the cot. When we put her in she screams and then we get complaints from the neighbours ... She knows the hostel. When I take her out, when we're coming back she just lies down in the road and screams. She doesn't want to come back.

So the child had been a source of worry to the mother for two months before the episode that led to a visit to the accident and emergency department. In addition, the mother explained that the child had a history of bronchitis – 'she gets it on the chest in the winter'. And she had been ill with respiratory conditions during the visit to Scotland. This is what the mother said about the illness for which she took Jean to the hospital:

She was very pale, and screeching, she wouldn't play with other children. She only ate in the morning and she had a runny nose. She was sick-looking in the night (*before*). I took her down the hospital mid-day. They examined her, they wouldn't believe she was sick. They said it was only a heavy cold. She looked really sick. I thought she had bronchitis. She kept clinging on to me. They kept saying why did you bring her down, why didn't you take her to the doctor? It put me off, with this bringing the child to the hospital. In Scotland she'd been very sick.

As the story demonstrates this mother and her family were living in stressful circumstances. The mother had long-term worries about the child's propensity to bronchitis and in addition felt the child was upset and possibly made ill because she missed her grandmother in Scotland and hated the hostel. So the mother thought any symptoms worrying and potentially serious. When the child fell ill one morning, she wanted help fast, faster than she could expect at the GP's, and in her view her action in calling the ambulance and taking the child to hospital was the best she could do for the child.

Discussion

Mothers' opinions of the health services and their accounts of recent meetings with health professionals show that they valued highly staff who took their perspectives seriously and made enough time to discuss children's health. It was notable that those who took their children to a specialist department of a hospital were particularly appreciative of this aspect of the consultation. Well-established good personal relationships with doctors and health visitors were important if mothers were to get the most out of the meetings. Most, but not all, the mothers had one or more 'good' health professionals to turn to. On the whole mothers thought they got a good service from staff, except that doctors – both GPs and hospital doctors – hurried the visit along, and some health visitors also rushed their visits. There was some criticism of the physical conditions in which services were offered – waiting rooms at GPs and hospitals were bleak and crowded, and some mothers said they had to wait far too long. Probably these problems relate mainly to stretched NHS resources. But where professionals behave as if they have too little time to give this may be partly because they do not know or do not recognize people's need for opportunities to listen and discuss.

Professionals' criticisms of parents for 'over-use' or 'inappropriate use' of services, suggest ignorance of parental perspectives. Parents do not go to the trouble of journeying with young children to the doctor or the hospital without good reason, as these mothers' stories show. They go because they need help and they are willing to put up with unsuitable waiting rooms and long waiting periods because of this overriding need. It is clearly inappropriate for professionals to remonstrate with parents when they ask for help. While it is understandable that service providers see a need to ration services, rationing should be done by planners and administrators, not by irritated doctors and nurses blaming individuals.

The study area provided services that were reasonably accessible, in the sense that they were there, if the customer was willing and able to go and get them, and to use another service if one was not open for business when needed. Mothers could see a GP within a day, in most cases. If not, they could take their children to a hospital. Getting a service from the GP at night was difficult and so mothers tended to take children to hospital then. Getting a home visit from the GP was difficult in a fifth of recent cases, and again most responded to this by taking the child to the surgery. Services that operate on the basis that people come to them rely on their ability to do so. Mothers with two or more children and no car may find that difficult – and delay could be dangerous for the child.

Were there class differences in mothers' use of services?

One of the study aims was to consider whether mothers all living in a small socially mixed area used much the same services and were equally satisfied with them. We noted that mothers in classes I and II were more likely than others to use group practices. A possible reason for this is that they said they particularly valued consulting a doctor who offered a 'paediatric' service, and this kind of differentiation of tasks is perhaps more likely in a group practice. But some mothers, especially 'local' mothers in classes III, IV and V, had been registered with the same doctor for several years, and some of these older, well-established doctors had not made the move to group practices. As for hospital use, the mothers used mainly the two hospitals nearest the study area, and equal proportions from all classes took their children to out-patient specialist departments and to accident and emergency departments. We cannot say whether use of specialist help was commensurate with need, but there were very few complaints from mothers that they failed to get help when they wanted it for their children. But mothers in classes III, IV and V were more likely than others to take suddenly ill children to hospital at night and at weekends. Numbers here are small (12 per cent in the last twelve months) but it was those with no telephone and those registered with one- or two-doctor practices who tended to do this. It is these doctors who most use the unpopular deputizing services. So it seems that these mothers had difficulties of access to their GP out of hours. Another reason for using the hospital was mothers' need for fast help with children who caused long-term worry, that is, persistently ill children.

There were few class differences in mothers' evaluation of services or in their satisfaction with encounters with professionals. Favourable and adverse comments on the GP, the health visitor, the developmental check and visits to the hospital came equally from all classes. But an important class difference was on the assessment of the health visitor's role, where classes III, IV and V were likely to see her as an inspector, and on the home visit by a health visitor, where classes IV and V found the visit intrusive.

We had no 'objective' means of evaluating the GP's service, but, judging by mothers' accounts, there were no class differences on some (relatively) factual points: journey time from home to the practice (though mothers with cars had easier journeys), waiting times at the surgery, doctor visiting at home in response to a request. This provides a contrast with Skrimshire's (1978) findings. She found that people in working-class areas were more dissatisfied with the GP service than those in middle-class areas, and they thought the poor service resulted from high case-loads and high need locally. As Skrimshire says, this still leaves open the possibility that doctors behaved differently to working-class patients (c.f. Cartwright, 1967). In our sample, mothers' accounts did not suggest such differences. But it is possible that some middle-class mothers had higher standards and better doctors whereas some working-class mothers had lower standards and worse doctors.

However, this sort of hypothesis seems unconvincing, considering that mothers' views on a variety of health services and professionals did not differ by class: the health centre generally, the developmental check, the quality of their health visitor and GP, the GP's practice, the GP's consultation, the visits to the hospital. It seems plausible to suggest that professionals were offering an even quality of service to different class groups. Several factors may be operating. Perhaps professional and maternal behaviour and interactions did not differ according to the mother's class, as others have found. Perhaps class III, IV and V mothers were benefiting by living in an area where good professionals worked. Perhaps mothers of all classes got a fairly even service because they were similar in their approaches to health care and to use of services, as we have suggested earlier. They were virtually all active and interventionist on behalf of their children's health and they wanted positive health for them (not just absence of illness). They seemed to use the services when they wanted to; they were not held back by deference or by other claims on their time.

Nevertheless, there was some evidence of class differences in access to health care. Mothers in classes III, IV and V faced more difficulties than other mothers in getting to see the doctor and some of them disliked the health visitor's role, as they perceived it. They also tended to use the hospital for emergencies, and though they tended to be satisfied overall with this service, it did involve them in distressing waiting periods and contact with harassed, sometimes critical, staff. Mothers' access problems can be linked directly to material disadvantages such as not having cars and telephones. These features of their perspectives on services and their use of services suggest a mismatch between maternal and professional views of services. If mothers distrusted the health visitors' motives and used the hospital 'inappropriately', they might be viewed by professionals as difficult customers and treated accordingly. Well-to-do mothers who did not feel threatened by health visitors and who could use hospitals in accordance with convention might, for these reasons among others, establish better relationships with health professionals.

10

Using Preventive Health Services

Introduction

Mothers make up their minds when to use curative services on the basis of their need for help, and on the whole professionals wait to be asked for help and give it willingly, though some may argue that mothers over-use or mis-use services. On the preventive side, professionals are more interventionist: they proffer services and issue invitations and appointments. Parents do not always respond, however, and the literature on preventive child health service use abounds in terms such as 'low use', 'under-use', 'non-compliance' and 'default', which reflect a professional or administrative view that parents know what professionals want them to do and should conform.

Research findings from the 1950s onwards on take-up of preventive child health services have consistently shown class gradients, with socially disadvantaged children taken less often to clinics, and first children taken more than subsequent children (see Blaxter, 1981, ch. 10 for review). The Child Health and Education in the Seventies (CHES) study of a sample from SW England and Wales found that social class did not account for differences, but their more sensitive measure, a social index, did. In the first three years of life, children from socially disadvantaged households were taken much less often than others to the clinic. On take-up of immunization, studies have again showed a class gradient. The CHES study showed a marked difference between socially disadvantaged children and the rest, according both to class and social index. Children from poor urban districts were especially unlikely to be immunized compared to children living in other areas (Butler, 1977). There seem to be few data on take-up of developmental checks. Perhaps this is because in studies relying on parental reports it has been assumed that parents find it difficult to distinguish between routine consultations and formal check-ups. Or, where data derived from clinic records, these may have been poor, or clinic attendance was deemed more important by researchers than developmental checks. We decided to ask about them because we knew parents in the area were invited to use them and we were interested in the extent of take-up of services offered.

Several studies have considered consumer perceptions of the preventive child health services and reasons for using or not using them. Steiner (1977) found that mothers appreciated the accessibility and relaxed atmosphere of health authority centres (compared to doctors' clinics). Buswell (1983) found that women turned away from the clinic to their own social networks after the first few months of the child's life; they no longer felt a need for clinic services. Graham and McKee (1980) found that mothers of young babies would use the clinic service if they felt it was an important service and not easily fulfilled elsewhere; also that some mothers were distressed by incidents at the clinic where they had been made to feel guilty, inadequate or embarrassed.

In this chapter, mothers' take-up of services is described and explanations for use and non-use considered. It is worth noting at the outset that we do not address the question whether advice sessions and developmental checks are effective in screening child populations. What we do ask is, given that there are such services, do mothers find them useful. The aim is to provide information that may help professionals who provide preventive services.

Usage of Preventive Health Services

The health centre or GP clinic

The 135 families all lived in an area covered by two district health authority health centres, which offered among other services baby clinic sessions to which parents could take their children for weighing, advice, developmental checks and immunizations. Most of the mothers had started off when the child was born using the district health authority clinic (81 per cent) and the rest had taken their child to their GP's well-baby clinic. Since that time, 33 per cent of mothers had changed clinics, mainly because they had moved house, though a few because they were dissatisfied with the service. Currently 85 per cent of the mothers thought of the health authority clinic as the place they went to for preventive health services, and 15 per cent the GP's clinic. The only class difference in all this was that mothers in classes IV and V were especially likely to have changed clinic because they moved house. This pattern of usage is different from that in other studies; for instance, Moss, Bolland and Foxman (1982) note that in an outer London borough 'middle-class' mothers tended to use the GP's clinic and 'working-class' mothers the health authority clinic. But the services in inner city areas are organized in ways that encourage usage of DHA clinics. Few GPs run their own clinics, partly because premises are cramped. Most health visitors are area-based, rather than based at GPs surgeries, so they encourage use of their clinic, and mothers know they can meet their health visitor there. And the health centres are within reasonable distance of all the mothers' homes, which may not be so common in less densely populated areas.

In this discussion the mothers' usage of the preventive clinic service is considered irrespective of whether the service used was at the health authority centre or at the GP's. This is because numbers were too small to differentiate and because usage as against non-usage seems to be the important issue. However, there was no difference in take-up of immunization, of checks offered, nor in satisfaction with checks, according to whether the mother used the GP's clinic or the District Health Authority (DHA) clinic.

All but one of the mothers said they had taken their children to the clinic in the first six months of the child's life. Most of the mothers said they had been many times; 54 per cent ten or more times and only 15 per cent fewer than five. Most produced their DHA baby books to check their memory. Like others (e.g. Graham and McKee, 1980) we found a class gradient in numbers of visits, with much lower use in class I than in classes IV and V. Possibly the difference stems from an extra load of ill health among children in classes III, IV and V, and from higher rates of working among class I and II mothers. However, the study did not aim to establish reasons for attendance in the distant past, but did aim to see if there was a consistent pattern of usage over time.

In the most recent six months, 65 per cent of mothers had taken their child once or more to the clinic. Almost all these visits were for weighing, check-ups or immunization. Only seven went to ask for help with illness – rashes, vomiting, a suspected allergy, a sticky eye. Some of course raised questions about the child's development during check-ups. Few mothers took their children more than once or twice to the clinic. There were no class differences in the number of visits reported, or differences according to the child's age. So for this sample, for this age-range of children, the familiar pattern of lower use by socially disadvantaged mothers had not been established.

It is interesting that few mothers used the clinic for illness, since it is sometimes claimed that such 'inappropriate' behaviour is common; and that mothers should recognize and respect the distinct functions of clinic staff (preventive and developmental) and GP (curative). Both Steiner (1977) and Hendrickse (1982) found high rates of requests for help with 'medical' problems at clinics. But their samples contained all ages of under-fives, including many babies, and mothers often need help fast for ill babies, and not just in surgery hours.

Mothers' reasons for not taking their children any more to the clinic were essentially to do with their growing confidence as mothers. Some said they knew the child was healthy and progressing well, and they did not now need reassurance. ('I found I didn't really need the support any more. I'm confident as a mother.') Mothers pointed out that when a child was young and your first, you need frequent help.

> I took him when he was small to make sure he was putting on weight. They get little ailments when they're small. After a while you seem to know what's wrong with them.

In addition, of course, some mothers' and toddlers' days were busier than they had been. Going to the clinic was no longer a good way to spend the time.

> I'm too busy to go up there. And I'd rather take him for a run in the park.

> It was nice when Robin was small, to have somewhere to go. Nice to get out for an hour or so. Now he's more of a nuisance at the clinic. I

have to spend my time chasing him. So it's not much fun taking him now.

The morning the clinic operates is the morning I'm at work.

So some mothers no longer felt the need for help from the clinic, and indeed there was a common feeling that the clinic was mainly for babies. Some mothers said staff had told them so. ('They said there's no need to bring him now he's older. He's not due to go till he's three.') Probably there was a reasonable consensus between mothers and staff that in most cases children did not need to be brought to the clinic except for check-ups once all concerned were reasonably happy with the child's progress, and the first months were safely past.

The developmental checks

These are offered at the district health authority (DHA) clinic at 6 weeks, 7 months, 12 months, 18 months and 24 months; and at the doctor's well-baby clinic, according to surgery staff, at 6 weeks, 7 months, 2–2½ years (as recommended by the Royal College of General Practitioners, 1982). In all, according to their mothers, 58 per cent of the children had had all the checks appropriate for their age and there were no class differences, either in take-up of each check, or in take-up of all the checks offered. The proportions of children taken for each individual check, according to their mothers, were as shown in Table 10.1. The proportions drop off for the older children, but all are higher than those found in other studies done in inner city areas.

Table 10.1 *Proportion of children taken for developmental checks at different ages (%)*

	6 weeks	7 months	12 months	18 months	24 months	N
This study	84	85	89	71	75	135
Nicoll (1983)	76	72	44	33	34	136
Bax, Hart and Jenkins (1980)	70	57	58	46	49	

Note: For this study we have taken into account children's eligibility by age. Children who attended a GP have been excluded for the 12, 18 and 24 month checks. The Bax, Hart and Jenkins' percentages are drawn from clinic records; no number was available.

This study relied on mothers' reports; the other two on clinic records. The figures given by Nicoll are from a study in Nottingham, and they show a very sharp decline in attendance at one year. Bax, Hart and Jenkins' figures show a similar but not so sharp decline for an area of inner North London. As always in this study, it must be pointed out that the sample for this study was limited to households with a first child, for whom attendance has generally been found to be higher. Ethnic minority and lone parent households were excluded; possibly some parents in these groups may use these services less.

The reported decline in attendance for check-ups after one year should perhaps be seen in the context of lower clinic attendance generally. If mothers get out of the habit of going to the clinic, a visit for a check will be something out of the ordinary, for which special arrangements or changes to routines may be necessary. In addition, after the first three checks, mothers may feel reasonably sure that their child has no abnormalities – congenital or developmental. And, again, some mothers thought they would notice any problem in their child.

> The first two (*6 weeks and 7 months*) were valuable. If something wasn't spotted when he was little (*at 6 weeks*) it might have happened in between. But after that I can't see the sense of it because if something was wrong I should be able to feel.
>
> (*The check*) was useful at six weeks, because I wanted reassurance, because I was concerned because he was premature. But later on I didn't need to know anything because I knew he was alright. I'm not worried about him developmentally. I didn't need to know what they thought.

Most mothers (70 per cent) thought the developmental checks were valuable, without reservation. It was good to be reassured.

> I can't imagine there would be, but there might be something I hadn't noticed – walking, eye defect. And it's nice to be told your child's healthy.
>
> It's valuable to have them test the hearing and sight and reflexes, and listening to her heart.
>
> It's cheering to hear she's getting on well. It gives you the doctor's point of view. It makes you *sure*. I like to know what the doctor thinks.

The checks were seen as providing a professional view of the child's progress and they gave a technical assessment of the child that the mother could not make.

However, nearly a third of the mothers (30 per cent), equally from all classes, made adverse comments about the checks. Some said the checks were poorly carried out, or done too hurriedly.

> At twelve months they did his hearing. But it was a bit noisy. A lot depends on how much noise there is going round. He didn't react. The doctor said, was I worried about his hearing. And I said, no. So he said well, we can assume he's alright. They're not very well carried out, not what I'd call test conditions. Very haphazard.

Or the tests themselves were seen as inadequate. ('It's very crude screening, I think.') Or they didn't give mothers enough time to talk with the doctor, to discuss how the child was getting on and to raise problems.

> Too rushed, not enough time to talk. I certainly wouldn't like him for a doctor for John. They're overworked, there's too many people. Last time we were the last people to go in. And it, it just didn't tell me anything. He tested her eyes, looked in her ears, tested her reactions. But it was all over in about five minutes.
>
> It's perfunctory. Casual.

Some doctors were described as insensitive to mothers or to children. Mothers felt they were excluded from what was happening:

> Last time we went, I asked her, 'Is that good?' wanting to know if he was progressing well. And she said, 'Yes' – off-hand, and it doesn't really tell you anything.

Children were distressed by sudden or repeated demands on them and didn't perform to order; then the doctor worried the mother by suggesting 'delay' or deafness.

> For the twelve months test, I had to go back twice. Because she wasn't cooperating. It's a silly test. Children are too young at that age to do what they ask them to – look at a little ball on a wire rod. I wasn't worried about her sight, but it was a nuisance. Yes, I did worry a bit at the time.

Or the doctor communicated a worry about abnormality.

> One doctor told me he had a big head and I ought to watch out for his growth. It frightened the life out of me. He said it could mean he's very clever or it could mean something else. I was very bothered about it. But I didn't wait around, because I was just moving house, so I went straight to the (new) clinic and told them and the doctor there said he'd never heard such rubbish.

As some of the comments quoted indicate (and there are other similar ones) mothers wanted to know if their child was healthy, but they also wanted to know if there was a problem. What was very worrying was when the doctor briefly shared with them a suspicion, or a slight suggestion that something might be wrong or might need to be monitored.

> There's something about the way they – they half say something and then they say, Oh, no, I think it's alright. It's as if they were thinking of referring the child and then not. And they don't explain what they were thinking about.

From the doctor's point of view it is obviously difficult to strike a balance between alerting the mother so that she will monitor the child and bring her back for a further check, and unnecessarily worrying her. There is no easy answer to this. But mothers appreciated having a full discussion so that they knew what was being done and why. They found it easier to cope with a possible problem if they felt they had had a full explanation and a chance to discuss it.

Apart from their views on the value of the checks, mothers gave reasons for not attending for a specific check. Some mothers (21 per cent) said they did not know, until we mentioned it, that a certain check was offered (only one mother said she did not know at all about developmental checks being on offer). Others (20 per cent) said they were busy or forgot, or else they were sure the child was fine and saw no reason to go (25 per cent). And 9 per cent said they were in the throes of moving house at the time of one of the checks.

A third kind of information was available from the study to explain take-up. This was information collected at other points in the interview, but which the mother did not refer to when we discussed clinic usage. First, analysis showed that one group of mothers used the clinic more than the rest – the mothers who had told us they did not have enough people to talk with about their children's health and welfare. They took their children more often to the clinic in the first six months of life and more of them had been in the most recent six months. Many more had taken the children for the most recent developmental check (58 per cent compared to 31 per cent of other mothers). Possibly these mothers went for consultation and reassurance about their children's health and welfare, whereas the other mothers had enough discussion with relatives and friends to reassure them, so they had less need of help and support from clinic staff. Secondly, consideration of events in the household around the time of checks showed that eight of the mothers had been heavily pregnant or had just given birth to their second child; and 18 of the study children had been seriously ill. These families belonged equally to all class groups. But in addition, 14 families, all from classes III, IV and V, had moved house. So, it seems likely that one kind of reason why mothers did not take their children for checks was because there were other more urgent health care matters on their minds. In addition, moving house, which can be disruptive in many ways, perhaps affected contact with the clinic.

All in all, it is clear from mothers' accounts of their usage and experiences of the developmental checks that they agreed with professionals on the importance of establishing that the child was developing normally and progressing well. But there were areas of disagreement, possibly of misunderstanding. Doctors and health visitors perhaps assumed that mothers knew what each check was for, agreed that the checks were offered for good purposes, and agreed that they should bring their children to the service offered. Some mothers reasoned that if they were happy with the child's progress and were confident there was no abnormality then there was no need for them to have the child checked over. It was their responsibility to decide what help to seek for their children as and when they saw fit.

It was also evident that there were some failures of communication between health professionals and mothers. A fifth of the mothers said they didn't know there was such and such a check. The main confusion was over the later ones – at 18 months and two years, and some of this confusion probably stems from the fact that GP clinics and DHA clinics offer different sets. This was particularly difficult both to remember and to cope with for mothers who switched from one type of clinic to the other. At a more general level, it seems that doctors and health visitors had not made out a good case for all mothers to bring their children for all checks.

Immunization

For children up to the age of those in our sample the immunizations offered are three shots of vaccine against diphtheria,

Table 10.2 *Proportion of children immunized against different illnesses, by mother's class*
% *of children*

Mother's Class	Triple (DPT)	Double (DT)	Polio	Measles	N
I	67	13	100	87	15
II	58	40	98	75	40
IIIa	69	19	92	81	26
IIIb	57	43	100	71	28
IV,V	42	54	89	58	26
N	78 (59%)	49 (36%)	129 (96%)	99 (73%)	135

Kendall's Tau C = r = −.11   r = .11   r = −.04   r = −.11
p < .05   p < .05   p < .07   p < .05
Number of children = 135.

whooping cough and tetanus (DPT), three against polio and one against measles. In the study area children go on three successive occasions during the first year of life for the DPT and polio vaccines and then at about 15 months for the measles vaccine.

At the time the interviews were done (1982) there was well established concern about possible dangers to children of whooping cough and measles immunizations. At the end of the 1970s the rate of immunization against whooping cough was below 50 per cent. Uptake of measles immunization (available since 1968) has never been great and has remained below 60 per cent (OHE, 1984).

Both parents and professionals have been uncertain what constituted contraindications (Hull, 1981); publicity in the press has been adverse and myths have abounded (Nicoll, 1985). In this difficult situation, it is generally agreed by professionals and by parents that parents are responsible for making the decisions (c.f. OHE, 1984). Some doctors and health visitors advise, others offer 'facts' and leave interpretation to parents.

Only half the study children (51 per cent) had had all the immunizations on offer. There was a class gradient, with notably lower take-up in classes IV and V. Almost all the children had three shots of the diphtheria, tetanus and polio vaccines. But fewer had the three pertussis immunizations (58 per cent) and the measles immunization (73 per cent).

It emerged from what mothers said about immunization that they thought the decision rested with themselves, or with them and the child's father. This feeling that it was up to them to decide was reinforced by some health visitors and doctors who offered information but made it clear that parents took the responsibility for the decision.

The decision was difficult and often agonizing. Parents felt they had to weigh up various pieces of information and advice. They threw into the debate every piece of information and advice they could muster. Some had knowledge about the incidence of whooping cough and measles from their experiences in their own families and in the neighbourhood and some therefore thought it unlikely that children would get these illnesses nowadays. Another kind of knowledge was about friends' and relatives' children who had been brain damaged by the immunizations, or alternatively had been seriously ill with the illnesses. Some had read about such cases in the newspapers, or seen programmes on the television. Mothers sought advice and information from relatives, friends, health visitors and doctors. Some read pamphlets available at clinics.

People cannot usually tell you where they get their ideas from and we did not ask mothers the source of their views on immunization. We simply asked why they did or did not have them done. One thing that is clear in the immunization controversy is that advice is not clear-cut. For instance, if parents read the available literature they will find confusing, imprecise, worrying and contradictory advice and information. This can be illustrated by reference to three popular sources of information available in 1982.

The Health Education Council's leaflet 'Immunisation' (undated, but available at the time of the study) on diphtheria, tetanus, whooping cough and polio says:

> When you take your baby to be immunised, ask yourself these questions:
>
> Is my baby unwell in any way?
>
> Is my baby being given medicines of any kind?
>
> Has my baby had any side-effects from any previous immunisations?
>
> Has my baby, or anyone in my immediate family, ever had fits or convulsions of any kind?
>
> If your answer to any of these questions is yes, or if you are unsure, talk it over with your doctor.

On measles, the HEC's 'Measles is Misery' (also undated but available in 1982) says:

> It's natural for you to worry about the possible side effects of measles vaccination. But the facts are reassuring. It is very rare for a healthy child to suffer serious reactions such as convulsions or brain damage. Your child is much more likely to suffer such reactions after having measles itself.
>
> Some children have a mild fever after being vaccinated; a few develop a rash which is not infectious. These usually occur about seven to twelve days after vaccination and last only a day or two. You should see your doctor if there is a high or persistent fever or there are obvious signs of illness.
>
> PRECAUTIONS
> The vaccine must not be given, or must only be given in a modified form, if your child or anyone in your family suffers from certain conditions. So make sure the doctor knows about:
>
> *any illness your child is suffering from at the time
>
> *any health problems your child or your immediate family have suffered in the past, especially problems like convulsions or epilepsy
>
> *any allergies your child suffers from
>
> *any medicines or drugs your child is taking
>
> REMEMBER
> Measles is misery. Ask your doctor about vaccination now.

Leach (1979, p. 475) strongly advises in favour of immunization and does not enlarge on the debate. On whooping cough, she says:

> If he is feverish or seems ill ring your doctor. The baby may be reacting badly to the pertussis (whooping cough) part of the triple vaccine in which case your doctor should know so that he can decide whether to leave it out of the child's next shot.

And on measles:

> A very few children suffer convulsions after the injection. If this should happen to your child remind yourself that such reactions are much more common during a full scale attack of real measles. Because of this very small risk, a child who has had feverish convulsions will not be given the injection. Be sure to discuss any such episodes with the doctor who is to immunize the child.

Jolly (1981, pp. 241–43) says, on the triple immunization:

> If your baby has a reaction – if he becomes irritable, especially if he cries inconsolably and in a different way from usual, or feverish or off colour – let your doctor know. He may then decide to omit the whooping cough component from subsequent injections, since this is the most likely to cause reactions.

and he lists contraindications:

> Your doctor needs to know if your baby suffered any brain symptoms at birth, such as may follow a delay in taking his first breath. He must also know if your baby or any near relative has ever had a convulsion. Either of these would lead him to omit whooping cough vaccination because of the increased risk of complications.

On measles, Jolly says:

> There is a small risk of convulsions following measles vaccination but this is less than the risk of brain reactions as a complication of natural measles. A child with a history of convulsions is at a greater risk of brain reactions. Consequently, the doctor will only recommend vaccination if he gives a protective dose of gammaglobulin at the same time. A family history of allergy is a contraindication to measles immunization because some preparations of the vaccine have been grown on egg to which the child might be allergic.

These three publications have a good deal in common. All aim, explicitly, to ensure high take-up of immunization. All the authors assume that the doctor will decide what to do for the child or will say what is best. The parents' role is to provide such information as they can to help the doctor. The doctor is presented as one who knows the pros and cons and will make the right decision. Parents can rely on his (sic) judgement. However, the list of points parents should remember to mention is likely to raise their worries about just why they should mention them. For instance, some may take it that an ill or 'unwell' child should not be immunized. The information given is vague, especially on what constitutes 'immediate' or 'near' relatives. Finally, none of the publications recognizes the understanding that most professionals and parents share: that decisions are up to parents, that they accept and welcome this responsibility and that they want and *need* detailed information to help them decide.

Among those mothers who had all the immunizations done for their children, the main reason they gave (91 per cent) was that they thought it was the best way, all things considered, to keep their child safe. The decision was taken in the light of the individual child's welfare. A few mothers (14 per cent) argued that they had them done partly because they were content to follow the clinic programme. ('It seemed right; he's meant to have them.') In other words, few abrogated their own responsibility to decide. And few (10 per cent) made any mention of the wider issues in favour of immunization – that the nation's children would be better protected if everyone had their child immunized. ('It was for protection, for his health. I think all children should be done, then no one would get the diseases.')

What reasons did mothers give for *not* having the immunizations done? First, whooping cough. There were two main reasons. Some mothers (18 per cent), equally from all classes, said they were unwilling to take the risk of long-term harm to the child.

> I was frightened because of the brain damage scare. But I wish I'd had it done. My husband said no because of the brain damage. I could still take him to have it done – they say there's going to be an epidemic.

Others said there was a medical reason why the whooping cough immunization should not be done; there was a history of convulsions in the family or there had been problems at the time of the child's birth.

> I didn't have the whooping cough for Mark because my sister had convulsions. The health visitor told me about the contraindications and I decided not to have it done. The doctor said I was being stupid. He said I was a complete fool not to have it done. When doctors are talking to you they're intimidating. But I stood my ground. I said I'm not having it done. And I walked out and I never went back.
>
> He's a child with a birth history and they advised against it. And I know a child who was brain damaged by it. So I didn't want it done.

Three children reacted to the first shot of the vaccine. Altogether 23 mothers gave a medical reason, and here there was a class difference: 40 per cent of mothers in classes IV and V, compared to 14–17 per cent of mothers in other classes. The numbers are small, but it is perhaps worth adding that the main class difference arises from the fact that mothers in classes IV and V more often reported epilepsy and fits in the family, compared to other mothers.

The number of children not immunized against measles was

Table 10.3 *Immunization and reasons for non-take-up by mother's class (%)*

Immunizations	I	II	Mother's Class IIIa	IIIb	IV,V	N
All done	67	53	65	46	31	69
Not all done:						
Medical reason[a]	26	6	15	14	31	23
Other reasons[b]	7	40	19	39	39	43
N	15	40	26	28	26	135

[a] Medical advice/reason; reacted to first injection (3 children), got the illness (5 children).
[b] Mainly unwilling to take the risk (24 mothers).
All columns sum up to 100%.

smaller (37), an insufficient number to consider reasons given according to class. The main reasons mothers gave were that the child had an allergy: 'she was allergic to eggs, so they didn't do it'. Or again, that there was a history of fits or convulsions in the family.

It is notable that of those who relied on a medical argument against immunization, two-thirds said a health professional had advised them against it. It seems that mothers are likely to form the view from their own experience and from talking to other parents that health professionals will advise against, in respect of a high proportion of children, and that many children, possibly including their own, are not suitable candidates.

Taking mothers' perspectives as a guide to why their children did not have immunizations done, a picture emerges of their worries and reasoning. This is summarized in Table 10.3.

Mothers at the extremes of the social continuum tended particularly to refer to the medical risks to their children. Indeed if those 23 mothers who gave medical reasons are excluded from the analysis, then there is no significant difference along the class continuum in take-up, although there are wide variations between class groups. High proportions of mothers in classes II, IIIb, IV and V had other reasons for not giving their children the full course, compared to classes I and IIIa.

The numbers are small and it would be unwise to speculate much further about why groups of mothers advanced different reasons for their decisions. The fact that medical reasons were advanced more by some groups does not necessarily mean that there were more people in those mothers' wider families who had certain conditions. As far as we know there is no class difference in the incidence of fits and convulsions (Ross, Peckham, West and Butler, 1980). It could be a chance finding, or it could be that some mothers in different class groups had different motivations for advancing medical reasons. Some well-educated mothers may have had good information about contraindications and have thrown it into their decision-making process. Some mothers, particularly in classes IV and V, may have felt it important to provide a reason that would convince the doctors, and may in addition have had thorough knowledge of the illnesses that had befallen members of their wider family. Other mothers may have felt they could rely on just refusing the immunization in the confidence that they could withstand a challenge to their view.

These suppositions led us to consider whether some groups of mothers might be particularly heavily influenced by scare stories and hearsay. On the perhaps dubious assumption that women with lower educational levels might be more likely to fall into these groups, we analysed take-up of immunizations by educational level and found that, within classes III, IV and V, mothers with lower educational levels were less likely than others to have had all the immunizations done. Two other factors, whether the family had moved house once or more in the child's life-time, and persistent illness in the child (according to our definition) did not relate to take-up.

Another factor, rarely advanced as a reason, also accounted for some non-immunization. Having asked mothers for their *reasoning*, we asked whether there were any *circumstances* that made immunizing the child difficult. A substantial minority – 23 per cent – said the children had been ill (mainly with colds) on the appointed date – either too ill to take to the clinic, or too ill for the staff to be willing to do the immunization. Analysis showed that only half as many of these children had had all the immunizations compared to children not reported ill (29 per cent against 58 per cent). Some children had been ill for two or more appointments. It seems that if appointments were missed because of minor illness, the staff and/or parents did not always ensure the child was immunized on a later occasion.

Discussion

Class similarities and differences

The most striking feature about clinic usage is that in important respects there was equal usage across class groups. The clinic offered help with the common problems mothers have with young, especially first, children and it was still seen as useful for many mothers especially those who felt poorly supported by friends and relatives. Most mothers still found developmental checks worth attending. This was especially so for those who felt they had insufficient people to talk with about their children, compare notes and decide just how normal they were.

So there seemed to be a feeling among mothers that the clinic performed a useful function. It was seen as a place to go for advice and information on development as well as for immunization rather than for help with ill children. Mothers made up their own minds whether the services were useful. Those with good social support used it little, and decisions against immunization were reached after consideration of many factors.

The main class difference was on immunization – and this difference was large. Less than a third of children in classes IV and V were fully protected, compared to two-thirds in class I. A variety of explanations have been proposed. One is that mothers believed that there were risks for their child because of histories of fits and epilepsy in the wider family. Another is that they feared immunization because of its rumoured dangers, but relied on the fits-and-epilepsy argument because it might be more convincing to doctors. A different kind of explanation lies in the educational level of the mothers. It may be thought that professional-type knowledge is more common among the more highly educated and that such knowledge would tend to influence parents towards having immunizations done. As with many findings in this study, it seems more reasonable to suggest that all these factors may be important, than to argue in favour of one.

Preventive services – using and providing them

At the beginning of this section it was suggested that what the study shows about mothers' health care of their young children at home provides pointers to what they were likely to want from the health services. They saw themselves as responsible for the child's health and would want recognition of this responsibility. They would expect high quality services which were easily accessible, flexible and responsive. They would welcome opportunities during meetings to acquire knowledge from professionals. The data on mothers' experiences and views of preventive health care services can be viewed in the light of these propositions.

Mothers' use of these services was guided in the main by their perceptions of what was the best course of action for their own child. They took the children for the early developmental checks to make sure all was well, but some then decided there was no good reason to go on taking them. Similarly the decision to have immunizations done rested on the child's interests. An important aspect of their wish to do well for the child seemed to be the need to be sure in their own minds that they had taken into account all relevant factors when making decisions; and that they had followed up any suspicion they had of a health problem. It was clear that mothers valued opportunities to learn from professionals. One criterion of a good developmental check was that doctors allowed time to explain and discuss what was happening, and time for mothers to raise topics of concern. Many mothers had taken into account professionals' views when deciding about immunization.

The mothers' accounts suggest that they had few problems using the services. They did not complain of difficult journeys, problems with the hours offered, or difficulties in making appointments. As far as we could tell, the services were satisfactory in these respects. And most mothers seemed happy without reservations about the developmental checks; they found them reassuring or informative.

However, there did seem to be a central characteristic of service provision which made for difficulties for both mothers and professionals. Clinic services were offered on the basis that it was for parents to decide whether to use them. But there was a slightly uneasy tacit assumption, held by both sides, that professionals thought parents should use the services. For the mothers, the problem sometimes was that they did not have enough information on which to base their decision. In some cases it seemed they did not know what the professionals' arguments were for using the services. Some might suspect they were being asked to act in certain ways without having good reason to, or even that a health professional's advice or behaviour concealed another purpose. Thus Mark's mother (quoted earlier) felt she had to stand and fight about immunization. She suspected the doctor was trying for unstated reasons of his own to get her to act against the child's interest.

Indeed there is a mis-match between the interests of the professionals and the mothers. The mothers are aiming for good health for their own children. The professionals are working for the benefit of individual children too, but they are also trying to screen and protect populations of children. They want to immunize high proportions of the area's children, in order to reduce the chances of epidemics. They want to identify congenital problems, hearing and sight defects and developmental delay and to do this may ask mothers of healthy children to bring them time after time, so that all children will be screened at the appropriate age. Where there is any doubt they will ask mothers to bring the children back for another test, or refer the child on suspicion. But from the mothers' point of view, the half-voiced suspicions of professionals and their emphasis on retesting or on referral can lead to worry, which in the end turns out usually to be needless, in respect of their child.

However, while the perspectives and aims of professionals and parents may differ, and while this may be inevitable, it does seem important that parents should have good access to information about what the services are for and why professionals think they should use them. As regards immunization many mothers said they did talk with health visitors and doctors and they thus acquired knowledge to act on. It seems most health visitors and doctors were willing and ready to give information and to listen to mothers' views and fears. But the fact that half the children did not have all the immunizations done suggests that there was room for more, or possibly better, discussion and information-giving. It is essential for this that health professionals themselves have firm guidelines which they trust, as for instance implemented in Nottingham (Nicoll, 1985). It is also important that both parents and professionals are made aware of the dangers resulting from diseases such as whooping cough and measles as well as of the remote dangers of immunization. As the Office of Health Economics (1984) discussion paper notes, few people nowadays have first hand experience either of the illnesses or of damage caused by immunization; information about both should be made widely available to counter this (fortunate) ignorance. This is not to suggest that people will all, or always, act on the basis of knowledge, rather than of fear. But on balance perhaps more of them will, some of the time. In any case, mothers wanted to know the 'facts', to help them make good decisions.

As regards developmental checks, it seems plausible that if health professionals want higher take-up they will be successful if they follow the guidelines suggested by mothers' accounts of what was good and bad in their experiences. Mothers wanted to know why they should bring the child for each check, that is, what were the purposes of the check at each age, and why it was important that these purposes be achieved. They wanted checks to be carefully carried out in a suitable atmosphere – especially a quiet, non-hurried atmosphere. They wanted due attention paid to the age, sensitivities and character of the child. They wanted time to discuss what the check revealed of the child's progress, and opportunity to raise any topics of concern to them (c.f. Williams, 1983).

Current debates on developmental checks among professionals turn on the questions whether the checks do in practice pick up problems and on how to increase take-up. Mothers' accounts suggest that they share some professionals' view that checks are sometimes not thorough enough and that they are irritated by requests to go on attending when the child is doing well. Nicoll (1983) and Polnay (1985) argue for fewer tests at standard ages and for more thorough tests, when called for by maternal and/or professional concern and the child's history. This seems a sensible improvement to the usual rigid universal system.

The last section of the book presents an overview of mothers' health care of their young children, and some discussion of ways in which parents and professionals can work together to give children good chances of good health.

SECTION E

Discussion

11
The Study Reviewed

This chapter starts with a summary of the main findings of the study and continues with a discussion of some important recurring topics in the book.

Preventive Care at Home

This book has presented mothers' approaches to health care and their health care practices for their children. The central concern was whether these approaches and practices varied by class, and if so what factors provided good explanations for such variations.

Perhaps the most striking finding overall was the degree of similarity between mothers, and this provides a basic and crucial setting for the consideration of their children's access to health. For we found that virtually all the mothers had high standards for health in children and saw the promotion of health and the prevention of ill health as dependent mainly on parental care. They thought factors outside parental control − such as luck, heredity or the physical environment − were relatively less important in determining health status. On safety, again virtually all the mothers were highly aware of risks to their children and indicated their concern in their detailed accounts of what they did to protect their children, and how they altered their care as themselves child developed. All the mothers thought of food as important for the maintenance of health and they all claimed that intervention to promote good dental health was appropriate now.

So far as general orientation towards child health care is

concerned our findings suggest that virtually all mothers, of whatever class background, were highly motivated, positive and interventionist. This adds up to an impressive picture of a responsible approach to preventive child health care.

Mothers' accounts of their preventive care practices also suggest that the vast majority, in all class groups, were interventionist. But their practices varied by class and a number of factors can be identified to account for this variation.

Almost all the mothers took active steps to safeguard their children against risks, using a variety of strategies, termed by us supervision, reliance on the child and preventive action. These strategies were chosen to suit the type of risk, the home circumstances and the child's stage of development. (The proviso to this is that a small group of ten mothers seemed to rely overmuch on supervision alone compared to other mothers.) Mothers thought safety care practices were affected by housing conditions, in that they could not make the housing safer, and our analysis too showed that those in particularly poor housing were most likely to feel powerless in this respect. There was also an association between poor housing and children being reported as developing potentially dangerous characteristics. Finally, poverty was related to low ownership of safety gadgets, and some mothers also said they could not afford such items as fireguards and safety gates.

Mothers gave positive reasons for food choice. They chose food for their children according to sets of ideas about what was relevant to food choice, notably health, family custom, children's preferences. The type of food, judging by 'yesterday's' diet, varied by class in important respects. Moving along the class continuum children had less fruit and vegetables and more sugar and fatty foods. Again, analysis showed that poverty was related to low intake of fruit and vegetables. It seemed that there was a more firmly held belief among the more highly educated mothers (irrespective of class for classes IIIb, IV and V) that sugar was bad for teeth. And a number of other factors provide partial explanations for aspects of the children's diets: poverty; mothers' rationales for food choice, in 'health' or 'family custom' terms; their views on when main meals should be; their daily round of tasks and events and the child's social life. The data also suggested that the view that obesity is bad for health was less widespread among class III, IV and V, than among other mothers.

On dental care, all mothers claimed to be taking some action 'now' — mostly restricting sugar and/or brushing children's teeth, and equal proportions by class, said tooth-brushing had taken place 'yesterday'. Again, there was a specific piece of knowledge that was referred to by more educated mothers (to some extent independently of class grouping): that is, that fluoride was good for teeth. And mothers in classes I and II, most of whom did have high levels of education, claimed to have carried out more dental care actions 'yesterday' than other mothers did. However, nearly half the mothers said something had affected their usual dental care behaviour 'yesterday'. Other health care priorities intervened, there were unusual events and crises, children and parents forgot, children refused to brush their teeth. Who brushed children's teeth, when and why at that point in the day varied widely. This may be because mothers did not have access to a firm and consistent body of knowledge about what kinds of dental care are appropriate. Use of dental care services varied by class, and it seemed likely, as others have suggested, that socially disadvantaged mothers were disadvantaged in this respect too, in that they themselves had poorer relationships with dentists.

The findings on preventive care at home suggest some explanations for differences in health care — differences that affect children's access to good health. These explanations are broadly material. Some households had poor material resources for giving their children good health care. Parents living in poor housing found it difficult to keep their children safe, low income affected parents' ability to give children good food. Mothers fortunate enough to have good levels of education had access to information about, for instance, sugar and fluoride, and this information may have helped them towards good nutritional and dental care practices — good, that is, according to current professional advice.

This study points to material resources as important factors explaining child care practices. In this respect it differs from many studies (mainly from the 1960s and 1970s) which argue that mothers in households suffering severe social and economic disadvantage bring with them from their own upbringing or acquire sets of behaviours which deviate from those of most mothers.[1] Such studies argue that some disadvantaged mothers are unwilling or unable to give active care to their children; they are apathetic in their approach to child care and afflicted with a sense of hopelessness and powerlessness which has a profound effect on their behaviours including their child care practices. More recently Blaxter and Paterson (1982) found among their sample of mainly class IV and V mothers in Aberdeen that the most socially disadvantaged had 'a disorganized and sometimes apathetic approach to preventive care'. In general, these mothers had low expectations of normal health and there was little evidence of a positive concept of well-being.

Perhaps three points can usefully be made about these research findings. First of all, most studies are about samples of mothers who are well advanced in motherhood. That is, they have several, or many children and are coping not just with financial, housing and marital problems but with the demands of many people in the household and the pressing need to do paid work outside the home. It is not surprising if mothers in these circumstances put preventive health care fairly low on their list of activities. By contrast we chose to focus on households where these extra burdens carried by many working-class mothers in the later years of motherhood had not yet descended with full force. Choosing to study first-time mothers of young children also allowed us to catch them with their ideas about optimal health and preventive care relatively unsullied by hard experience and conflicting demands on their attention.

The second point of difference between many such studies and ours concerns reasons and purposes for doing the studies. Many studies start with a model of how mothers should behave and seek to identify behaviours that 'explain' why mothers do not conform to the model. For instance, some seek to provide explanations why mothers do not use preventive services for themselves or their children. They start with the view that mothers are 'poor utilizers' and attempt to identify poor features of their practices at home which then are used to support the view that the women are poor mothers. The view that low usage reflects poor mothering generally is very prevalent (see e.g. Jones, 1984). Some studies are within the casework tradition of social work. While recognizing that material circumstances may be important in affecting behaviour, they seek to identify behaviours which may be modified through social work intervention, as one means of helping people in difficult circumstances. At the root of problem family studies, particularly, is the view that individuals' behaviour can change or be changed without altering the material circumstances in which they live, desirable though that might be. However, in the present study we started not with the proposition that something was wrong or poor about mothers' approaches and behaviour, but with the aim of identifying what those approaches and behaviours were. We sought understanding of mothers' care at home and how they perceived health services. Probably this difference goes some way to explaining differences in findings.

The third distinctive feature of the study was that we focused on mothers' opinions and behaviours almost exclusively in connection with the child. Other studies of women's health beliefs have considered the topic generally or have put together what they said about both adults and children.[2] As suggested in Chapter 5, it may be that mothers' perspectives on optimal health and the causation and prevention of illness are different for adults and for children. They may have higher standards for children. This is to argue not that people's basic ideas about health will vary depending on whether they are thinking about adults or children, but that they may think more can and should be achieved for their children.

It is being suggested here, in fact, that we focused on the 135 mothers at a particularly good time, when they were through the early worries of first-time parenthood, but not overwhelmed by the burdens that for working-class mothers become heavier as time passes. As mothers of first young children they had in common their 18 months or more experience of working for their children's health. Mothers in all class groups were able to rejoice in their active, playful and investigative toddlers, spoke about these qualities with pride and were willing and able to work to maintain their children in this healthy state. This was so even among those mothers who lived in some of the worst circumstances. While explaining problems of coping with their children in poor housing on low incomes, they still described enthusiastically their children's high activity levels and abounding interest in the world around them.

That is the general picture. However, two points need to be made about it. First, most health professionals and social workers know of mothers who seem not to give the same high level of care to their children as the vast majority do, because of their health or preoccupation with other concerns – such as, their career or financial or personal problems. At a very impressionistic level, we felt this kind of unease about two or three of the 135 mothers. They came from both 'high' and 'low' class groups. Professionals may wish to intervene in such households to safeguard the children, but such cases do not constitute a basis on which to construct a theory that many mothers are inadequate parents, or even (a current trend) that parents in general need to be taught how to parent.

The second point is that, even within the children's narrow age-range, there was some evidence that as the children grew older mothers in the poorer households were finding it more difficult to care for their children well. For instance, mothers in classes III, IV and V were particularly likely to think their children were developing potentially dangerous characteristics, and from a younger age. In another year or two it might seem to an onlooker that the children had been inappropriately or poorly socialized. There was also some evidence that within these same classes children at the top end of our age-range (30–36 months) were having a poorer diet than younger children. And there was also a pointer to increasing class divergence in dental care as children got older, in that among the older children it was mostly those from the top end of the class continuum who had been taken for preventive check-ups.

The important finding is that mothers across all class groups started off with much the same ideas about children's health and much the same aims, with the primary objective to keep them healthy. But as time went on, class differences in practices appeared and these can be linked to material resource problems. For instance, children in poor housing were especially difficult to manage. Controlling types of food intake became more difficult as children got older and entered a social world where sugary and fatty snacks were the norm.

The general conclusion must be that if we are concerned to intervene to improve children's access to health, then judging by this sample of mothers we would do well to build on mothers' good qualities and opt for improving their material circumstances, so that they can care for their children's health as they wish.

Caring for Ill Children and Using Health Services

Sections C and D of the book consider mothers' care of ill children and their use of health services, both curative and preventive. Chapter 8 is an exploration of patterns of *mothers' care of ill children*. We found that a quarter of the children (27 per cent) were persistently ill and they came mainly from households in classes III, IV and V which had particularly poor resources for child rearing. The mothers of these children had serious long-term worries about their children's health and they tended to seek medical help more often and faster than other mothers, especially if they also had poor social support. So the study suggests that it is important to consider mothers' use of medical help in the context of the child's health history and the mothers' social support system.

A second major point to emerge from the study of recent illness episodes was to do with knowledge. Some mothers did not know whether to contact doctors, many did not diagnose illness correctly (according to the doctors' diagnoses) and many went to the doctor at least partly to increase their knowledge. Mothers acquired knowledge through the experiences of child health care, from doctors and health visitors and also from their friends and relatives. Those with poor social support (predominantly in classes III, IV and V) lacked this important source of knowledge.

Finally, we learned from accounts of recent illness that there were various constraints in the care of ill children. Many resulted from the complexity of interacting events and commitments within households – such as adult illness, paid work and housework problems, and problems caring for younger siblings. In addition, poverty and poor housing led to difficulties, mainly for classes III, IV and V.

In Section D mothers' perspectives on and use of services were explored in the light of their approaches to health care at home. It was suggested that they would wish health professionals to respect their wishes and value their knowledge; and that they would have high standards for services; they would expect flexible responsive services; and would value opportunities to discuss their children's health and to learn from professionals.

Mothers' views on GPs and health visitors and their accounts of recent meetings with health professionals showed that they did value professionals who were pleasant and thorough in their work, who respected mothers' views and knowledge and gave enough time to discuss the child's condition fully. Mothers were willing to tolerate poor waiting conditions and long waiting periods provided they got this kind of service from doctors in the end. They were correspondingly dissatisfied when professionals hurried the meeting or criticized their behaviour as parents.

In the main, mothers perceived health visitors as having a supportive, responsive role. Most were happy with the interventionist side of the health visitor's job. Home visits were mostly perceived as useful. But some socially disadvantaged mothers felt the threat or had experience of unwelcome and unacceptable intervention in their lives.

Apart from this, study of use of services showed some class differences. Class I and II mothers were more likely to use group practices. Access to services was more difficult for class III, IV and V mothers and some mothers living in poor circumstances, and with doctors offering a poor out-of-hours service, tended to use services rather differently from others – they took their children without appointments to the hospital.

Chapter 10 considered perspectives on *preventive child health services*, again in the light of the data on health care at home. Mothers used clinic services if and when they perceived them as useful. Usage of the clinic had dropped off since the first six months of life, and mothers' acquired confidence in their knowledge and abilities as mothers seemed to account for this. As with care for ill children, it was those with poor social support who particularly sought help from clinic staff. Mothers felt responsible for their children's health and for deciding whether to have developmental checks and immunizations done. In the case of immunization they weighed up what they knew, sought advice and took the best decision for their children. Data on both check-ups and immunization suggested, again, that they valued opportunities to discuss their children, and to acquire knowledge. There were no class differences in reported recent usage of the clinic or in take-up of developmental checks. But there was notably low take-up of immunization in classes IV and V. On the general assumption that better knowledge would lead to take-up of immunization and that education gives access to knowledge, it is interesting that those with the lowest educational qualifications in classes III, IV and V were unlikely to have had the immunizations done. And children ill at the time of appointments were also relatively unlikely to have completed the course compared with other children.

During this exploration of mothers' health care of their children at home and their perspectives on services, some topics have recurred. The rest of this chapter draws out three of these – knowledge, control and responsibility – and considers what light they throw on mothers' behaviour and how they help in considering relationships between parents and professionals.

Knowledge

A recurrent topic in this study has been what mothers know and how their knowledge relates to their health care practices. Four sorts of knowledge are distinguished here for the sake of clarity, though in practice they merge into one another.

First and foremost, mothers knew their children, and so they were sensitive and responsive caregivers. They modified their health practices to suit the child's mood or health status or developmental stage. A mother who perceived a child needed comforting gave her a treat – perhaps sweets or crisps; if the child looked ill or tired, she would alter her diet or abandon toothbrushing for the day; she would balance restricting the child against letting her explore, depending on her perception of the child's safety-consciousness and reliability. To put it another way, mothers were engaged in various kinds of health care for their children; with the emotional, social and developmental needs of the children as well as with physical health. In addition, of course, they were concerned with the welfare of all household members, so that care of the child took place amid other priorities: the emotional, social and health needs of siblings and adults. Mothers had to decide when it was necessary to draw on and concentrate all available resources into caring for the child. Indeed the accounts of crises, accidents and sudden acute illness stand out in the interviews partly because they were occasions when many resources – parents, relatives, professionals, transport and medical technology – were mobilized and concentrated on the child's urgent need.

Thus the study throws light on an important point: maternal health care of young children is a delicate balancing act which depends on mothers' knowledge and judgement. Those of us looking on can trust mothers, because in important ways they do know best. But for mothers in poor material circumstances giving children good care was difficult because so many factors constrained their behaviour. Intervening in this complex world, for whatever reasons, must be carefully done if it is to be acceptable and effective.

A second sort of knowledge mothers have comes under the broad umbrella of 'lay' health knowledge, that is, the body of knowledge that the mothers brought to bear on child care: acquired since childhood, supplemented, modified and deepened through the experience of child care, through reading and through discussion with friends and relatives. It provided a basis for action in the case of minor illness, safety care, nutrition and dental care, though mothers often wanted to supplement or replace it with a medical opinion.

Two interesting points that seem to have been important for health care emerged from this. One concerned social networks. Mothers in classes I and II – who tended to be satisfied with the quality of support they had as regards caring for their children's health and welfare – frequently discussed minor illness with relatives and especially with friends. So they had good access to this source of knowledge. Mothers in classes III, IV and V used this source less for illness, probably partly because many had more seriously ill children, and also because some felt they had insufficient people to turn to. So these mothers turned to the doctor for help and perhaps relied more on doctors' help than class I and II mothers. It was also notable that poorly supported mothers used the clinic more than those who had plenty of people to turn to. And lonely mothers with serious long-term health worries about their children needed a lot of help from professionals. Our data do not allow us to speculate whether these frequent contacts led mothers to acquire knowledge that helped them care for their children. But the data fit in with other studies which suggest that mothers of chronically ill children tend to be dissatisfied with the quality of professional help. Perhaps this dissatisfaction arises partly because, whatever their access to 'lay' advice and knowledge, they need more time and discussion with professionals than most give.

The other point of interest was floated tentatively in Chapter 5. It seems important to discuss it briefly here. There were two rival structures of thought about the maintenance of health. Put schematically, giving the two ends of a continuum, on the first view it was important to *ward off* attacks of disease. Children should be kept warm – warmly dressed, warmly fed, possibly fairly fat – and dangerous substances should be cleaned off the teeth. On the second view it was important to *build up* a child's resistance to ill health, including dental ill health, through diet and dietary supplements (vitamins and fluoride). One approach to the explanation of mothers' nutritional and dental practices is through examination of this continuum and where they stand on it. In support of this tentative thesis it can be said that among class III, IV and V mothers there was more expressed concern with hygiene and with keeping children warm; mothers gave their children more sugared and fattening foods, but also took action to clean the teeth. At the 'top' of the class range, mothers talked more than others about how food promoted health and prevented illness; they also gave their children better food (but there could be other reasons for this, as suggested in Chapter 6); and they claimed to try to build up children's teeth.

It has been suggested along the way that their expression of these views and the fact that they claimed to act on them relates to their good access to some of the messages professionals would like us, the population, to absorb and implement. Broadly these messages concern daily preventive practices to improve our health. So this is a third kind of knowledge some mothers possessed. Using educational level as a crude indicator of access to this kind of knowledge we found it was indeed the case that more highly educated mothers whatever their class tended to voice opinions and refer to practices that fitted with these professional messages. Given that those at the 'top' of the class continuum almost all had high levels of education, unlike most of those at the 'bottom', there was in effect a class divide. Mothers in classes III, and especially in classes IV and V, were relatively unlikely to talk in terms the professional would approve. This raises the question of health education, which we take up in the next chapter. Here it is worth saying that given mothers' commitment to doing their best for their children, there seems no reason to suppose they would be unwilling to learn and change their behaviour.

Indeed it was clear that mothers sought to hear professionals' perspectives: their views and knowledge on specific health care topics of concern 'now' to the mothers. This is a fourth sort of knowledge. Thus, notably, the mothers aimed to get professionals' views on immunization when they were trying to decide what to do about it; during developmental check-ups they wanted full discussion of the child's development and of suspected incipient or possible problems; during consultations with doctors for illness they wanted a professional diagnosis and, again, discussion of the seriousness of the condition, how to recognize it, what to do about it. They asked health visitors their opinions about matters to do with pregnancy and new-born babies; they valued hearing their opinions and advice on housing, marital and adult health problems.

So mothers turned to professionals partly to learn from them. They had a certain respect for the professional view and actively sought to hear it. Some clearly thought that doctors would, or even should, hold a clear view on specific topics. But mothers also knew from experience that for some problems in child health care doctors and health visitors had no specifically professional knowledge to impart. And they knew that individual doctors and health visitors varied in their views and some were better informed than others.

These points support our impression that mothers sought the professionals' knowledge in an open-minded way. They viewed it, not as ultimate or unified truth, but as educated opinion. They took it seriously as one important kind of knowledge, to be used alongside the other kinds they possessed when making child health care decisions. And as the data suggest (Chapters 9 and 10) they did not all, always, think they had enough opportunity to hear and discuss professionals' views. The point is taken up in the last chapter.

Control

This study pointed to wide differences in resources between mothers, broadly as grouped by occupational class, and it was part of the purpose of the study to explore whether and if so how mothers' health care practices were affected by the resources they had. Whatever kind of health care was considered it was clear that while most mothers in all class groups had similar aims and equally serious approaches to health care, poorly resourced mothers were hindered in their practices.

Well-to-do mothers had a high level of control over the way they did their health care work, because they had enough suitable resources, such as housing, income, cars and phones and help with child care. To summarize, most of the mothers in classes I and II were in housing owned by the parents, had moved in before their first child was born, had enough money to alter it to suit adults and children; could get about by car; ring for help; keep up social contacts by telephone and car; earn money themselves and pay for help with child care. It has been argued in this book that these resources allowed them to put into practice what they aimed for in health care to a far greater extent than poorly resourced mothers could.

This contrast was the more striking because all the mothers were, in important respects, similarly placed – with a first child and another adult in the household. And it has been noted that there were already hints that as life became more complex – as the child grew older, the social and neighbourhood environment became more salient in her life, a second child was born – good child care became more difficult for mothers. And it would become much more difficult for poorly resourced mothers.

To hypothesize, as children grow older one would expect poor housing of the kind described to make adequate safety care almost impossible. For example, Harrison (1983, ch. 16) describes the difficulties Hackney mothers of primary school children had in safeguarding them in dangerous estates and neighbourhoods. Children's diets will contain more and more sugar and fat as the children join a social world where such a diet is usual, and as household resources are more tightly stretched to provide adequate food for older and more people. Getting children to health services will be increasingly difficult if there are several children *and* no telephone and no car. Forced mobility as parents struggle to obtain appropriate housing is likely to continue to disrupt social networks, make it difficult to use local health and child-care facilities, and increase the burden of child-care work carried by women. Of course, when these factors are combined the burdens may be overwhelming.

It was noted earlier that the idea of a 'culture of poverty' has been popular among many commentators, including people in the caring professions, to explain what are seen as deviant or inappropriate behaviours by people living in extremely deprived and stressful circumstances. Also deeply engrained in public and private thinking is the idea that there are broad class differences in child-rearing ideologies, in aims and practices. Distinctive patterns of working-class child rearing have frequently been documented and explored, to inform middle-class readers and to endorse ways of life unfamiliar to them (e.g. Hoggart, 1958). In addition there seems to be widespread support in Britain for the view that personal characteristics rather than structural factors account for poverty. For instance, a 1975 EEC survey on people's explanations for the causes of poverty found that the British were far more likely than the French, Italians or Germans to opt for individual laziness and lack of willpower as explanations in preference to 'injustices in society', 'bad luck' or 'the inevitable price of progress' (Jones, Brown and Bradshaw, 1983, ch. 10). The two strands – two cultures defined by class, and individualist explanations for failure – run together, to produce the deeply held belief among middle-class people, including professionals, that working-class people have different aims, behave differently, and are less virtuous than themselves.

Perhaps the most influential and thorough-going attempt to contrast middle-class and working-class child-rearing practices has been Newson and Newson's longitudinal Nottingham study (e.g. 1965, 1970, 1978). Their aims, procedures and conclusions are important just because the books have been so widely read and are the most complete account available of child rearing in Britain. To take their study of four-year-olds (1970) (the nearest age group to that in this study): it selected 700 children randomly from the city's birth records, omitting single and 'immigrant' households and those with handicapped children. Each child's mother was interviewed. There were, as in our sample, large class differences in housing conditions. Working-class families mostly had four or more children, while middle-class families mostly had one or two. The study children could be first or subsequent children, and obviously their chances of being second or third children were much greater in the working-class families. The Newsons identify large class differences in child-rearing practices. These are sometimes discussed and explained in terms of housing or numbers of children. But parity is little used as a distinguishing factor and given the evidence (c.f. Dunn, 1984, ch. 6) that parents do rear first children differently from subsequent ones, parity would probably have explained some important differences. Again, with hindsight, the relevance of poverty to child-rearing practices might perhaps have been considered more carefully. And the combined effect of several, probably adverse, factors is not considered. The main thrust of the book is to describe class differences and then to identify, explore and elaborate different underlying ideologies of child rearing.

Working-class ideologies and practices are seen as inferior to middle-class ones. The expressed belief is that while material circumstances may affect or even determine some practices, child-rearing ideologies persist and survive environmental improvements.

The work done for this present health study provides a useful perspective on the Newsons' work. It suggests the importance of recognizing how seriously parents' practices may be affected by their environments. It also draws attention to the value of distinguishing between approaches and practices. It calls in question, at least for the health-related branches of child care, the notion that there are very different, class-related, ideologies at work. Both the Newsons' work and this study suggests that middle-class mothers had much greater control over their lifestyle and their child-care work than working-class mothers. While possibly, as they suggest, there may be broad differences in child-rearing ideologies, we would argue that on health care, mothers have essentially the same aims and preferred methods.

People who provide services to mothers of young children are as likely as anyone else to assume that they differ by class in ideologies and day-to-day aims, and that their practices reflect these underlying forces. These are understandable assumptions, given the literature and prevailing modes of thought. It is suggested here that such assumptions need to be carefully considered. At least as regards health care it is probably more appropriate and effective to deal with people as individuals and to take into account their circumstances and their level of control over their practices.

Responsibility

Study evidence is that mothers took a responsible attitude to child health care and to use of services. In a sense this is obvious and everyone would agree that they do. Mothers know that they feel responsible for their child's welfare. Professionals who deal with mothers and children also know that mothers carry the responsibility for their children – for supervision, for decisions, for welfare. And wherever mothers turn they are reminded that everyone assumes so. The message is beamed at them by advertisements for soap powders and baby foods, by health visitors and doctors, nursery school teachers and social workers; and by public policies on taxation, maternity benefit, day care for under fives and education. All suggest that mothers are ultimately in charge.

At the same time, however, there is an important strand in public and professional thinking which assumes that mothers, or some mothers, do not take enough responsibility for their children and that it is one of the tasks of professionals and policymakers to urge them and help them to do so. This view has a long history. The provision of services for mothers and babies developed in the early years of this century in the context of concern about high rates of child mortality and morbidity. While material circumstances were seen as relevant factors, maternal ignorance and irresponsibility were identified as key factors too. And action was directed mainly at mothers rather than at poverty. The provision of clinics ('schools for mothers') and of home visiting schemes was made with the specific aim of monitoring and improving mothers' health care of their young children (Lewis, 1980). The view that people should take more responsibility for their health became a particularly important theme in government thinking during the 1970s and can be seen in the context of the crises faced by health services as they failed to conquer the major health problems of industrial societies, and faced concurrently increasing demands for health care and increasing restrictions on expenditure.[3]

A series of DHSS papers was issued stressing prevention as the way forward in health care and the 1977 White Paper 'Prevention and Health' summarized the departmental view.

> Much ill-health in Britain today arises from over-indulgence and unwise behaviour. Not surprisingly, the greatest potential and perhaps the greatest problem for preventive medicine now lies in changing behaviour and attitudes to health. The individual can do much to help himself, his family and the community by accepting more direct personal responsibility for his own health and well-being. A principal aim of 'Prevention and Health: Everybody's Business' and the associated series of preventive follow-up papers is to remind the public that this responsibility is everybody's business and that it is in everyone's own interests to adopt a healthier style of living.
>
> (para. 131)

As regards child health care, the 1977 document referred back to earlier reports and agreed with them that a change was needed both in parents' and professionals' role in child health care. It will be noted that when discussing the care of children the documents refer to 'parents'. Substitution of the word 'mothers' and then of 'fathers' is an interesting exercise (c.f. Graham 1979).

Health surveillance in pre-school and school years
The Sub-committee referred to the need for regular health checks, and the Court (1976) and Brotherston (1973) Reports stressed the role of health surveillance for all children. They discussed its importance as a means of monitoring development and as an opportunity for health education and helping parents to understand their role in looking after their children's health. They thought that professional staff should regard parents as partners with them in the care of their children rather than as passive bystanders; this has significant implications for professional training.

(para. 105)

The 1977 suggestions were taken up by the Royal College of General Practitioners (RCGP)in a report on 'Health and Prevention in Primary Care' (1981). This identified the GP and the primary health care team as the appropriate professionals to encourage preventive care. One of the GP's functions was to help patients (sic) take responsibility for their health. The problem was to get people's cooperation: 'Many people still believe that responsibility for their health can be left to professionals' (Chapter 4). For instance, getting children immunized was a problem for health visitors: 'For them, registers, reminders and invitations are essential tools, justified the more because not all parents are fully informed or fully responsible about the care of small children' (Chapter 3).

A second report from the RCGP (1982) focused specifically on preventive care services for children. This report took up the challenge presented in the 1977 report (quoted above, para. 105); it is a particularly important report here because it considered the division of responsibility between parents and professionals for children's well-being. In the first five chapters, the report identified constraints affecting child health: the environment, including the home; and deficiencies in services. It proposed the primary health care team as the most appropriate system for providing child health care services. It discussed the role of surveillance of children and how to provide it; and considered the organization of the practice and of the team. The report went on in Chapter 6 to discuss a new relationship between doctors and 'patients'. It argued that doctors should become more active than they had been traditionally; instead of waiting to be asked for help they should intervene to promote certain kinds of behaviour, particularly in relation to preventive medicine and with reference to children and old people. Two measures were proposed as regards children. First, doctors should 'take the initiative', by sending for 'defaulting' children to be surveilled and immunized, and by opportunistic health promotion – teaching prevention when people attended for other purposes – such as for help with illness. Secondly, doctors should keep good records of the children registered with them in order to see that all were covered by these preventive activities.

But, the report argued, if doctors changed their orientation to provide a higher profile service, 'patients' must also change.

> If the primary health care team is to increase its activity and responsibility, this must be balanced by correspondingly increased activity and responsibility on the part of patients especially parents and children, who must increasingly accept responsibility for their own health. This responsibility can usefully be classified as follows:
> 1. The responsibility of being informed:
>   (a) About the skills needed to rear children, the importance of their emotional and physical environment, and the risks to their health.
>   (b) About what preventive care is currently available.
>   (c) About medical services and how to make the best use of them.
> 2. The right to question.
> 3. The right to refuse.
> 4. The responsibility to work with primary health teams.
>   (Royal College of General Practitioners, 1982, ch. 6.)

If 'patients' were not to become 'the helpless playthings of the professionals' they had 'a duty to be informed by society and by the professionals of the latest information in health fields'. 'Patients' must recognize that they could do more than ever before to maintain and improve their own and their children's health. Primary health care workers should help them assume this responsibility and should be willing to discuss, explain and inform.

Such willingness (to discuss, explain and inform) on the part of health professionals is just what the mothers in this study appreciated, and the more of it the better. They needed full information on preventive services and why professionals thought them valuable. And as we have suggested earlier, mothers sought the opportunity to learn what professionals thought on a wide variety of health issues, both curative and preventive, so that they could make informed decisions. So the RCGP's proposals here are welcome. Further, as the report says, if doctors take a more interventionist line, it is crucial that people should be well informed and confident so that they can hold their own and retain the ability as well as the right to make their own decisions. The concept of a partnership between professionals and parents, where both bring knowledge to the task of ensuring children's good health seems eminently acceptable. So far, so good. But this report, like the earlier one and the DHSS 1977 White Paper, relies on several contentious arguments.

First, it is suggested by the RCGP that primary health care teams at GP practices should provide preventive care for children, and should keep adequate records of coverage (c.f. Stacey and Davies, 1983). The difficulty here is that while a GP's practice may reach complete coverage of those registered, this by no means ensures that all children in an area are monitored and covered. Area-based services must continue, particularly in inner-city areas with mobile populations.[4]

Secondly, the RCGP assumes that if health professionals provide certain services and urge people to use them, people should fall into line. That is they assume consensus on the superiority of professionals' knowledge and orientation to service use. But this consensus does not exist. People do not agree that professionals know best. Indeed the RCGP's concept of a partnership surely encompasses recognition by both sides of the knowledge and serious approach to health matters of the other's side. Furthermore, people know there are varying views among professionals. For instance on developmental checks, mothers know GPs and clinics offer different sets; on immunization they find that professionals' knowledge and practice vary.

Thirdly, the reports, while paying some attention to material factors as they affect health, see individual behaviour as likely to affect health, independently of material environment. This is perhaps not very surprising. Health professionals deal with individuals and intervene to promote good health at the individual level. To think in individualistic terms is appropriate in their daily working lives. But professionals and policy-makers also propose that general explanations for poor health lie with individuals' behaviour. This is an increasingly popular view at present. Of course, it is an attractive view because to aim for changes in individuals is cheaper than to tackle poverty. In addition, present Conservative Party ideology promotes belief in the power and duty of individuals to shape their own lives. It is not suggested here that it is useless for individuals to change their behaviour, only that it is more difficult for those who are socially disadvantaged to do so, and that the positive effect of such changes may be small compared to the adverse effects of material disadvantage.

Finally, of course, the DHSS and the RCGP argue that people do not take enough responsibility for their own health, that is, they act in ways that jeopardize their own and their children's health, and they rely overmuch on professionals to keep them healthy. Professionals should foster a sense of responsibility in their 'patients'. The argument presented in this book is that if mothers do jeopardize their children's health, it is unknowingly or because they lack the power to do otherwise. And this study, like many others, suggests mothers certainly do not rely on doctors to keep their children healthy. Indeed almost all the health care children receive is given by mothers. They know it is up to them to care for their children's health and they see the services as helping them in that task, when they see fit or need professional knowledge, skill or treatment.

Notes to Chapter 11

1 e.g. Philp (1963); Tonge, James and Hillam (1975); Wilson and Herbert (1978). See also Lewis (1963) for the original formulation of the concept of cultures of poverty and Jones, Brown and Bradshaw (1983 ch. 10); Coates and Silburn (1970 ch. 7) for commentaries.
2 Pill and Stott (1983); Herzlich (1973); Blaxter and Paterson (1982).
3 The topic has been considered for the United States by, e.g. Crawford (1977) and for the UK by Graham (1979).
4 As the Court Report (1976) and others say, e.g. Bax, Hart and Jenkins (1980).

12

Helping Mothers Care for Their Children's Health

Introduction

The study described in this book was undertaken in order to contribute to explanations for class inequalities in health. Its specific contribution is in exploring processes which affect young children's access to health, and to health services, through examination of their mothers' care: mothers' beliefs and approaches to health care, their practices and factors that affect their practices. The study focused on a sample limited to certain sorts of households and it focused on some specific topics within the broad field of child health care. It was concerned with one, important, aspect of health – children's access to health – and with one, limited, sample, in one area of London.

The descriptions of mothers' health care given in this book should be viewed in the context of other findings on inequalities in health in childhood over the years and, notably, as reviewed in the Black Report (1980). The data lend support to the two-pronged approach suggested by the committee to reduce inequalities: improving the material environment in which children are reared; and finding ways to improve services provided for young children.

In this chapter some comments and suggestions are made for ways forward. These derive from the study – though they are not strictly confined to it. They rely to some extent on the large-scale statistics – for instance on accidents or dental health, to which reference has been made. The discussion here is at a general level;

it is not appropriate in the aftermath of this one study in a large field to make detailed prescriptive suggestions for policy-makers and practitioners. First are some brief notes on resources for health care, and second a discussion of ways in which professionals can help parents care for their children's health.

Improving Resources for Health Care

This study has suggested that *poverty* constrained mothers in their health care. Purchasing good food and safety gadgets, making the home safer, contacting health services for help, all were more difficult on low incomes. As has been graphically described elsewhere, parents cannot rear their children well at current rates of state benefit (e.g. Burghes, 1980). Poverty in childhood is a major national problem. Recent studies have suggested that a third of under-16s are now being reared in households which cannot meet basic subsistence needs (e.g. Piachaud, 1981b). The findings of this study support the argument put forward in the Black Report (1980): the reduction of poverty may be desirable in principle; as a matter of expediency, the poverty of households with young children must be tackled if we want to see reductions in health inequalities. They suggest as the main strategies the index linking of child benefit *and* an infant care allowance paid to mothers of under-fives. The Black Committee is assuming the status quo: mothers, not fathers, carry the work of child care and need resources to do it. Of course this division of labour by sex is not immutable. It is a matter of political will to offer fathers incentives and opportunities to care for their children. Some have argued for income maintenance on the Swedish model – the payment of a high proportion of 'normal' wages while a parent (either sex) stays away from that work to do the work of child rearing (see discussion, Moss 1985).

The poverty of many households with young children is a condition parents cannot individually tackle while levels of *pre-school provision* remain so pitifully low. Virtually all care for under-threes is in the private sector; it is scarce and expensive. Childminders offer the largest number of places; there are very few nursery places, and only well-to-do people can afford in-house help. The childminding service is variable and often poorly supervised (Mayall and Petrie, 1983) and is unpopular with parents. For over-threes the situation is somewhat better. Though most care is part time (in local education authority classes and schools and in playgroups) and there are still not enough places, it is free or cheap. The upshot is that parents with under-fives cannot, unless they command high salaries, both choose to go on working full time. An expansion of properly monitored, cheap day care is urgently needed, so that parents may choose how to arrange paid work and child care to suit individual household members.

At present policy on pre-school provision in Britain assumes that choosing to use it is a private matter and that state intervention is inappropriate except for about one per cent of under-fives deemed to be in 'need' of day care. It is assumed that most parents will arrange for one of them (the mother) to stay at home with the children. This is a deficit model of pre-school provision, relying on the notion that a young child will be harmed by separation from her mother. We ought in Britain to take into account the well-established principles and practices of many European countries in perceiving pre-school experience as positive for young children, and as one means of enabling parents to choose how to arrange their lives. But there are other good reasons for urging the expansion of pre-school places. Children in inner-city housing need the opportunity to spend part of the day in more suitable surroundings – with space to play safely indoors and out. Children everywhere benefit from mixing with their peers. In addition parents rearing their children in poor housing need a break from their children, if they are to go on giving good care.

Inner-city *housing and neighbourhoods* are prejudicial to the safety and well-being of young children. They are both dangerous and constrictive of normal childhood activity and exploration. As the Black Report says (Townsend and Davidson 1982, ch. 9) it is remarkable, given the large, recurrent toll of accidents to children, that so little has been done to separate traffic from children. And it was distressing in our study to find that some of the newest housing estates in the borough were designed so that children could easily fall – off balconies, down stone steps and through open tread stairs – and that they had inadequate space indoors and none outdoors. Some of this was probably due to cost-cutting and the urge to build high-density housing. Some is thoughtless design. As Sinnott (1977) notes, architects award each other prizes for design features which people find dangerous in practice.

We endorse the Black Report's recommendation that coordinated policy should be formulated and implemented – for instance by the Health Education Council and the Royal Society for the Prevention of Accidents – to improve children's environments, by keeping safety issues (and we would add *health* issues) at the forefront of the minds of planners and architects.

Measures to provide parents with an environment conducive to effective health care should include coordinated *food policy*. Mothers faced many pressures to give children fattening and sugary foods. Restricting sugar totally was almost impossible. National changes in dietary attitudes and habits are needed, so that such foods are no longer an important part of the diet. There are welcome signs that some such changes are under way. The NACNE Report (1983) on nutritional guidelines for health education was taken up by the media and recently there have been many newspaper reports and TV programmes about diet; some manufacturers and supermarkets are promoting 'healthy' foods; food labelling slowly improves. But nationally promoted policies are necessary too, as with smoking, to discourage some foods, by taxation and by publicity. It was noted earlier (Chapters 6 and 7) that it is unrealistic to expect individuals to win against the food industry; national and large-scale changes are more likely to be effective. As Downer (1984) points out, the improvement in children's dental health in the 1970s (see Todd and Todd, 1985) probably resulted from large-scale changes, as well as from individuals' behaviour. Fluoridation of water supplies in some areas and the adoption of fluoride by toothpaste manufacturers were important. Some baby food manufacturers began to produce sugar-free or sugar-reduced foods. Vitamin supplements were produced in drop form, instead of in sweetened syrups. And mothers gave children less sugar in bottles and comforters.

Finally, there is the matter of *education*. What mothers told us about health care demonstrated that health care is a complex job. It demands sensitivity to the child, attention to family patterns of behaviour and individuals' needs, the application of knowledge, and constant learning on the job. These were abilities and skills mothers displayed as they talked. In addition, they are asked by professionals to be quick to learn from often brief consultations and to adopt new approaches and practices. To get good quality help they need to be able to present their case. There seems little doubt that people who are used to collecting and interpreting information will, on balance, be well placed to acquire knowledge and to communicate with professionals. These skills are among those children learn through the experience of general education at school. For very many reasons it is advantageous for both girls and boys to stay in education beyond the minimum age, and especially so that they can live an independent life. If part of women's – and men's – adult life is spent rearing children then educational experience may be an important factor in helping them do it well.

The health care of children is viewed by professionals and media people as an important parental task, to judge from the amount of advice offered – though offered mainly to mothers. Health education literature, moreover, urges adults to care for their health. However, this literature sometimes gives simplistic messages and is individualistic in approach – it downplays the material realities of people's lives and the constraints that affect their capacity to choose certain behaviours (c.f. Farrant and Russell, 1986). If people are to take the maintenance of health seriously it is important to start with children and to interest them in health issues. Yet, apart from programmes aimed mainly at altering behaviour, more general health studies are little promoted in schools. 'Non-academic' girls may do a child-care course. Other children – boys and 'bright' girls – are rarely asked to think about health. But it could be an important school subject for all children, of all ages. 'Health' could cover topics such as health beliefs and practices; social, occupational, and geographical inequalities in health; and health service systems. It is a subject readily lending itself to a multiethnic and international approach. It has obvious day-to-day relevance and significance in children's lives. It can be studied from both theoretical and practical angles. It allows links to be established between school and real life, for safety officers, nutritionists, doctors can be brought in to school, and children can be taken out to study aspects of health in the locality – in supermarkets, housing estates, clinics and factories. A welcome move has been the development of an Open University course on health. This work could be extended to cover school-age children.

Professionals' Dilemmas

People in the caring professions have a particularly difficult task at present. Within services they face cut-backs, with loss of staff and reductions in the quality and quantity of what they can offer. Concurrently the people they serve are themselves seeing cuts in important services: fewer day-care places, cuts in housing programmes, closures of local schools and hospitals. State benefits fail to keep pace with the cost of living. And high levels of unemployment seem here to stay for the foreseeable future. People 'in the community' are having to care for the young, the old and the handicapped with poorer services to call on, and on smaller household incomes.

Professionals stand at the interface between services and people, and it is clear that in the present climate they are finding it necessary to reconsider what kind of service they should and can give. The debates concern the principles underlying the services, and where the services should pitch themselves on certain continua.

universal	---	selective
responsive	---	interventionist
structural	---	individualist

Health professionals are currently debating whether they should aim to cover everyone (in the practice, in the area) or whether they should concentrate scarce resources on a few, judged to be in particular need because, for instance, they are economically or socially deprived, perceived to be poor copers, or ignorant, or at risk for health or behavioural reasons. Similarly, should professionals wait to be asked for help or should they offer it and indeed propose lines of behaviour? How far should they operate on the basis that only structural or societal change can level up people's ability to manage well and achieve good health, and how far should they try to relieve difficulty and suffering in the here and now and work to change people's behaviour?

As noted earlier (Chapter 11), the Royal College of General Practitioners (1982) has responded to the problem of inequalities in child health with an essentially individualist approach. They suggest a programme of opportunistic health education of parents (mothers) by doctors. The proposal aims for universal coverage, on the basis that almost all children come with a parent to a doctor – for cure or prevention – at least once a year. So the doctor is seen as offering both a universal and interventionist service. The proposal rests on various assumptions: that parents, not doctors, should spend time journeying and waiting; that parents will agree that doctors' knowledge is superior to their own; and that they can implement doctors' suggestions, given their social and economic circumstances. In the end, it is seen as very much up to parents whether they are 'responsible' enough to attend, and to do what they are told. However, the report also argues that doctors should occasionally visit the home in order to learn about the child's environment.

But, this is by no means the only response of the medical profession. For instance, it has long been recognized that services must be planned to suit the social and economic circumstances of people in a given area. Doctors have provided evening clinics, and made home visits for developmental checks and immunization to children whose parents do not bring them to clinics. At a more general level the recognition by doctors that environment does affect health has led to the argument that the medical profession should press for environmental change (see for discussion Chalmers, 1985).

What constitutes an appropriate service for the 1980s is of particular concern to health visitors. Traditionally theirs is a supportive service whose strength lies in its universalist approach. Routine visiting has been acceptable to mothers because it is universalist. This universalist approach, together with emphasis on one-to-one meetings in people's own homes has made it an expensive service. However, as this study has suggested, the interventionist side of the health visitor's work is problematic. While some health visitors may think it part of their job to encourage certain sorts of behaviour, some parents may find such intervention intrusive and unacceptable. Other health visitors believe that health education aimed at individuals is less likely to be effective in improving health than community work aimed at giving people knowledge and power to change their circumstances.

Moreover, another factor has entered the equation. Pressure is growing for health visitors, like other professionals in the health services, to account to management for what they do and to justify their daily activities. Increasingly, the health visiting profession is questioning whether it can and should continue to aim for universalist service in the face of social problems, the pressure for accountability, and inadequate staffing levels. Should health visitors, like social workers, concentrate on problems? And if health visitors do that, will they remain acceptable, responsive and perceptive health workers?

It is an important principle that health services remain universalist in approach. Giving and asking for help to restore and maintain health should be seen as normal and useful activities. At a practical level too it is important that health services remain universalist, while offering a flexible response to individual need. Only so can people's sense of responsibility for their own and their children's health and their confidence in their knowledge and ability to carry out health care work be maintained. The alternative to a universalist approach is a selective one based on the judgements of professionals. This gives a dangerous amount of power to some groups of people, who are as prejudiced and limited in their views as anyone else. It is likely to undermine people's confidence in asking for help and to encourage victim-blaming by professionals. A selective service is unlikely to be effective in supporting and enabling people to give themselves and others good health care. In addition, if health services become selective there is a real danger that, as with other selective services – such as the day nursery – they may fail to meet need.

How Professionals Can Help

Resources

First and foremost people in the medical and community nursing professions can urge governments to put greater *resources* into primary health care services and into 'the community'. So-called community care can be a workable, effective reality only if people have resources adequate to the task of caring for the young, the old and the handicapped. The Black Report (1980, chs 8 and 9) argued for increases in staffing levels in community nursing, the family practitioner service and in school health services, and for increases in welfare foods and in pre-school provision. This study endorses the need for more staff time to be made available to parents, and for food policy to comprise action rather than just exhortation. Research work on pre-school provision in the context of the lives of households with young children supports the Black Report's recommendation that local authorities be obliged to ensure adequate day-care provision in their areas (c.f. Hughes *et al.* 1980).

Some of the problems with services our mothers (like others) met, can be solved mainly by better staffing levels. Mothers needed access to professional help on a 24-hour basis, and needed to be assured that someone would visit at home if need be. These needs can be to some extent met by reorganizing work and by forming groups of professionals to cover on a rota basis. Health visitors might consider providing a drop-in service at the clinic as a partial alternative to a home-visiting service. But there seems little doubt that existing staff levels are perceived by health professionals as inadequate to meet these needs. Usage of hospitals for emergencies could be reduced (with benefit to staff, children and parents) if primary services were perceived by parents as totally reliable. Mothers' wish for full discussion about their children can be met only if staff do not feel harassed and pressurized by staff shortages, though staff can also be trained to behave at meetings as if they are willing and able to give enough time to each person.

Partnership

Secondly, the findings of this study suggest that professionals can help by implementing the concept of *partnership* with mothers in health care. It has been suggested that professionals should recognize and respect the health care work of mothers, their responsibility for their children, their wish to discuss adequately the child's health and development and to hear the viewpoint of professionals.

Practical partnership between mothers and professionals has a number of elements. Perhaps most important it requires professionals to listen to mothers and to learn from them; to seek to understand their beliefs and aims and the circumstances in which they rear their children. In our multiethnic society this need to learn is particularly urgent. Listening and learning is important not so that professionals are better able to teach mothers (parents) what they believe to be true and useful – though that is a relevant role – but so that they can modify their own beliefs, aims and understanding of the context of child rearing. Professionals can also (and this is not contradictory!) provide *opportunities for mothers to learn*, to ask about particular problems and to discuss issues, such as immunization, developmental checks, respiratory conditions and behaviour problems.

Some recent initiatives in health care provide useful pointers to ways in which opportunities for learning on both sides can be provided. Health visitors are increasingly using group discussion as a means of opening debates about issues of current concern to mothers. Doctors and dentists could do this too. It may be useful for a range of people from different disciplines and with differing perspectives to discuss issues together. For instance dental officers and dentists, mothers, teachers, doctors and community nurses could usefully consider together dental health and initiate practical programmes to improve health locally.

The above suggestions are made in the context of current reality: it is mothers not fathers who in the main do the work of child care and take the day-to-day decisions, including whether to use services. Health professionals on the whole work with this reality: by directing publicity and by organizing services (e.g. clinic sessions are in the day-time) towards mothers, not fathers. Many fathers feel unable to take much responsibility for the care of their children, given the widespread acceptance of the traditional sexual divisions of labour. Health professionals cannot on their own do much to alter this situation. But pressure by parents and acceptance by professionals has brought about a marked change at the point of childbirth: many fathers are now present for at least part of the labour. Health professionals should perhaps consider how they can help to involve fathers in childcare work and child-care decisions, for instance by directing publicity and information towards fathers, and by pressing for parental leave from paid work for both fathers and mothers to see to their children's health needs.

Parents and others 'in the community' are forming groups themselves to discuss health issues, their health needs and how far local health services are useful to them. Such groups may wish to invite health professionals to contribute. Group work of this kind can supplement individual contacts between people and professionals; it can deepen knowledge and widen perspectives on health issues. Self-help groups have been important in affecting (indeed, improving) services, for instance for children in hospital. It is important for health professionals to be receptive to 'grass root' perspectives.

Another important way of recognizing in practice the concept of partnership and the primacy of the parental role is by the giving of *information*. To take the case of immunization: it has been noted (Chapter 10) that baby book and Health Education Council advice is inadequate, misleading and may be unnecessarily worrying. Given that parents have to make the decisions there seems to be good reason to give them access to the information professionals have, for instance the handbook given to medical and nursing staff in Nottingham. Similarly, parents could be given much fuller written information than is usual on developmental checks: what each check covers and why it matters. This sort of openness is likely to lead to better understanding and trust between professionals and parents, and probably to higher take-up. Finally, the parents' responsibility for the child can be recognized by giving them the *child's medical records to hold*. This has been done for many years in France and has recently been implemented in Oxfordshire. It is appropriate for parents to keep this information for they need to know for future reference the names of professionals who treated their child, the dates of treatment and the advice given; and they can spot discrepancies and inaccuracies. Furthermore, they can keep it all together, whereas current practice ensures fragmentation of any one child's records in various offices, filing cabinets and print-outs. Parents do not, contrary to some professionals' expectations, lose their children's notes. This system also has the advantage of tilting the balance of knowledge and expertise towards parents: at each meeting it is professionals who have to turn to the parent as the major authority on the child's health history.

Partnership with parents involves, as suggested here, a variety of means of sharing the care appropriately. It also demands that professionals provide *a service that meets the standards of parents* and is thus acceptable. This point has practical implications.

Our study showed that mothers wanted professionals to have detailed knowledge about child development and child care, to be sensitive to children's needs and behaviours during meetings and to respect their views as mothers. These findings lend support to the views of others on the child health services. It has been noted that many doctors who carry out checks at clinics are not paediatric specialists and may not offer a service to match parental wishes (Bax, Hart and Jenkins, 1980). In some areas health visitors run many of the clinic sessions (MacFarlane and Pillay, 1984) and also carry out many of the tests, especially sight and hearing tests; it is argued that doing these in the natural surroundings of home may improve the accuracy of the testing. What is important is that training for work with parents and young children should be adequate at both a technical and personal level to enable all staff to give a satisfactory service.

Health professionals should also provide a coordinated and coherent service. People approaching any one health professional should be able to get consistent information about the services. Thus doctors and health visitors at a health centre should be clear what each thinks about immunization and if individuals differ should be aware of these differences and be able to tell parents about them. Doctors and health visitors should know what local dentists think about dental care and service use. So health professionals in an area need to work together as a team in order to exchange information and coordinate service provision. The concept of team work is in turn leading to gradual acceptance of the idea that joint training courses or joint core training should be provided for all professionals who deal with parents and young children.

Finally, it should be said that the message coming through to professionals from mothers is on the whole an appreciative and understanding one. The services are perceived as useful, indeed vital; the constraints professionals work under are taken into account. But health professionals can do themselves and young children good by pressing for better resources in the community and in the health services and by taking serious account of mothers' perspectives.

Appendix

Mother's Class

In this study we wanted to be able to relate our findings to those of other studies, most of which have used father's occupation (Registrar General) as the social class indicator. Yet we also wanted to take into account the mother's part in influencing the life-style of the household and we were particularly interested in using an appropriate discriminator when considering mother's opinions and behaviour in looking after her child's health. We could use her own main past occupation as another measure, but this had the disadvantage that the women fell mainly into two large groups – those in class II jobs (professional workers) and those in III non-manual jobs (office work and shop work). This division did not provide for fine enough discrimination between mothers. We decided to use mother's education as a measure and this provided a good discriminator on its own. In this education measure we have amalgamated academic qualifications and training, since academic qualifications alone do not account for the varieties of educational experience of many women:

Mother's education

Group 1 – degree or further degree, or training as teacher, nurse, social worker or for other jobs classed as RG I or II (N–51)

Group 2 – 'O' levels or 'A' levels (N–26)

Group 3 – training for RG III non-manual or manual work (N–17)

Group 4 – no qualifications above CSE and no training (N–41)

The division is based on the assumption that the grades represent different levels of access to the written word and so to ideas. In practice the definitions and ordering did discriminate mothers in rank order, on levels of knowledge and types of belief. Of course education and training is closely related to class origin – a point discussed in Chapter 3.

For some purposes, where it was important to retain comparability with other research, but also to build in recognition of the mismatch between fathers in III manual work and mothers who were in III non-manual work or had relatively high educational levels, we devised a grading of households, which we called *Mother's Class*. The fathers in jobs classed III were divided into two groups:

1. where the father was III non-manual, or where the father was III manual and the wife had 'O' levels or above (i.e. she was in Group 1 or 2, on educational level).
2. where the father was III manual and the mother had no qualifications above CSE (i.e. she was in Group 3 or 4).

The choice of dividing points between the four grades was made on the assumption that reaching them *demands differing levels of application*. In this sense, among others, the four grades represent different education levels.

TABLE A.1 *Fathers' occupation (Registrar General) by mothers' educational level*

N (col %) Mothers' Education	I	II	IIIN	IIIM	IV,V	IV
Group 1	14 (93)	31 (78)	1 (11)	5 (11)	0 (0)	51
Group 2	0 (0)	6 (15)	4 (44)	12 (27)	4 (15)	26
Group 3	1 (7)	1 (3)	0 (0)	12 (27)	3 (12)	17
Group 4	0 (0)	2 (5)	4 (44)	16 (36)	19 (73)	41
N	15	40	9	45	26	135

Kendall's Tau C = .62; $p < .001$.
(*Note*: the 13 unemployed fathers have been recoded according to their previous (in all cases, main) job.)

Table A.1 shows how class III was divided up. The 26 households in the L-shaped box became class IIIa and the other 28 became class IIIb.

The use of Mother's Class thus allows for discrimination by mothers' education in the middle of the occupational range, but broad comparison with the Registrar General's classification is still possible.

Tables for Appendix

Some additional tables that may be of interest are given here. Note that all the information derives from interviews with mothers.

TABLE A.2 *Number of mothers/occupational class distribution of interviews by father's occupation (Registrar General) (main sample)*

	I	II	IIINM	IIIM	IV and V	Total
Mother interviewed	15	40	9	45	26	135(82%)
Family moved	2	1	0	6	8	17(10%)
Mother refused	0	2	3	5	3	13(8%)
Total	17	43	12	56	37	165(100%)

TABLE A.3 *Age of childen*

	\multicolumn{5}{c}{Focus child's age at interview (months)}	
	Under 18	18–23	24–29	30–36	37–40	N
Number	2	51	31	49	7	135
Percentage	1	38	23	33	5	100

TABLE A.4 *Proportion of mothers who said they carried out any preventive health actions against colds or illness generally (%)*

Mother's Class	\multicolumn{3}{c}{Any preventive health action}	
	None	For child only	For child and self	N
I	0	7	93	15
II	10	20	70	40
IIIa	15	8	77	26
IIIb	21	32	46	28
IV,V	11	38	50	26
N	17	30	88	135
%	13	22	65	100

All rows sum to 100%.

TABLE A.5 *Proportion of mothers who said no action was possible against falls inside dwelling by Mother's Class (%)*

Mother's Class	No action possible	Other answer	N
I	13	87	15
II	10	90	40
IIIa	23	77	26
IIIb	43	57	28
IV,V	31	69	26
N	32	103	135

Kendall's Tau C = $-.23$; $p < .01$.
All rows sum to 100%.

TABLE A.6 *Number of dangerous and unalterable features of housing mentioned by mothers, by tenure (%)*

Tenure of dwelling	Number of features				
	0	1	2	3+	N
Own	53	28	17	2	53
Not own	27	29	24	20	82
N	50	39	29	17	135

Kendall's Tau C = $.34$; $p < .001$.
All rows sum to 100%.

TABLE A.7 *Children's consumption of fresh fruit and vegetables 'yesterday' by household income (%)*

Household's net income	Number of portions of fresh fruit and vegetables consumed 'yesterday'				
	0	1	2	3+	N
Less than £100	53	29	0	18	38
Over £100	23	22	23	32	87
N	40	30	21	34	125

Kendall's Tau C = $.23$; $p < .001$.
All rows sum to 100%.

TABLE A.8 *Mothers' reasons for food choice by Father's Class (% of mothers)*

Father's Class	Reasons				
	Health only	Health	Family custom	Family custom only	N
I, II	47	96	53	4	55
III, IV, V	21	87	79	14	80
All mothers	32	91	68	10	
N	43	121	92	14	135

TABLE A.9 *Timing of child's main meals by Father's Class (%)*

Father's Class	Mid-day	Mid-day and Evening	Evening	N
I, II	59	20	20	49
III,IV,V	13	17	70	75
N	39	22	63	124
Total row %	31	18	51	100

All rows sum to 100%.

TABLE A.10 *Proportion of mothers who said they tried to restrict sugar, by Mother's Class (%)*

	I	II	IIIa	IIIb	IV,V	N
No	20	18	23	50	46	42
Yes	80	82	77	50	54	93
N	15	40	26	28	26	135

Kendall's Tau C = $-.28$; $p < .001$.
All columns sum to 100%.

TABLE A.11 *Number of sugared items consumed 'yesterday' by Mother's Class (%)*

	0–2	3,4	5,6	7+	N
I	21	36	7	36	14
II	32	32	14	22	37
IIIa	19	35	15	31	26
IIIb	0	18	25	57	28
IV,V	12	23	19	46	26
N	23	37	22	49	131

Kendall's Tau C = .18; $p < .01$.
All rows sum to 100%.

TABLE A.12 *The 350 illness episodes mothers reported for their children*

Respiratory and ENT		Skin conditions	
Cold (including chill, runny nose)	72	Rash (unspecified)	18
		Eczema	9
Tonsillitis (including sore throat and throat infection)	23	Nappy rash	8
		Stings, bites and abrasions	5
Earache/ear infection	19	Impetigo	1
Cough	13		
Bronchitis	6		41
Flu	4		
Chest infection	3		
Croup	1		
Wheezing	1	*Genito-Urinary*	
Asthma	1	Vaginal infection	2
		Tight foreskin	2
	143	Urinary tract infection	1
		Penis infection	1
			6
Gastro-intestinal			
Stomach upset (including stomach ache, vomiting, gastroenteritis and constipation)	26	*Teething*	
		Other	
Diarrhœa	23	No diagnosis specified	23
Loss of appetite	12	Virus, bug, germ	8
		Nothing the matter	8
	61	Combination	3
		Fever	2
		Irritable hip	2
		Eye infection	2
		Verucca	1
Diseases of childhood		Cold sore	1
Measles	7	Inflammation	1
Mumps	1	Lack of food	1
Chicken pox	1	Reaction to medication	1
		Failure to put on weight	1
	9		
			54

No. of episodes = 350.

TABLE A.13 *Number of episodes of acute illness among children with and without persistent conditions, during the last three months (%)*

Persistent condition	Number of episodes of acute illness						
	0	1	2	3	4	5	N
Absent	1	22	39	25	10	3	98
Present	0	8	16	24	41	11	37
N	1	25	44	33	25	7	135

Kendall's Tau C = .38; $p < .001$.
All rows sum to 100%.

TABLE A.14 *Number of mothers who reported contacting the doctor on the first day symptoms occurred*

1. Mothers of persistently ill children

Satisfied with social support	First day contacts		
	None	Once or more	N
Yes	15	6	21
No	3	9	12
N	18	15	33

($x^2 = 7.7; p < .01$.)

2. Mothers whose children were not persistently ill

Yes	25	27	52
No	4	8	12
N	29	35	64

($x^2 = .85$ no significant difference.)

TABLE A.15 *Mothers who mentioned constraints on caring for their children when they were ill, by Father's Class and by whether child was persistently ill (%)*

Class I and II	Constraints mentioned		
	Yes	No	N
Child is persistently ill			
No	65	35	45
Yes	55	45	10
N	35	20	55

$x^2 = .07$ d.f. 1. No significant difference.
All rows sum to 100%.

Class III, IV and V	Constraints mentioned		
	Yes	No	N
Child is persistently ill			
No	54	46	53
Yes	86	14	27
N	52	28	80

$x^2 = 7.1$ d.f. 1 $p < .01$.
All rows sum to 100%.

TABLE A.16 *Proportion of children immunized: this study compared with national figures*

	This study 1982	England[a] 1981
Diphtheria	92	84
Tetanus	92	83
Whooping cough (pertussis)	58	45
Polio	96	82
Measles	73	55

[a] *Source*: DHSS (1982) Health and Personal Social Services Statistics for England, London: HMSO.

(*Note*: these represent completed courses (three shots for diphtheria, pertussis, tetanus and polio; one shot for measles).)

TABLE A.17 *Proportion of children who had all immunizations done according to whether they were ill for one or more appointment (%)*

Child ill for appointments	All immunizations done		
	Yes	No	N
Yes	29	71	31
No	58	42	104
N	69	66	135

$x^2 = 7.85; p < .01$.
All rows sum to 100%.

TABLE A.18 *Number of children who had all immunizations done by mother's educational level, for classes III, IV and V*

Educational level	All immunizations done		
	Yes	No	N
Group 1 (high)	3	3	6
2	13	7	20
3	8	7	15
4 (low)	14	25	39
N	38	42	80

Kendall's Tau C = .24; $p < .05$.

Bibliography

The bibliography is of works consulted during the writing of this book. Not all are referred to in the text.

Acheson Report (1981) *Primary Health Care in Inner London: Report of a Study Group* (London: London Planning Consortium).
Barton, M. (1979) 'The idea of race and the concept of race' in G. K. Verma and C. Bagley (eds) *Race, Education and Identity* (London: Macmillan).
Bax, M., Hart, H. and Jenkins, S. (1980) *The Health Needs of the Preschool Child* (Report to the Department of Health and Social Security unpublished).
Benson, S. (1981) *Ambiguous Ethnicity* (Cambridge: Cambridge University Press).
Blume, S. S. (1983) 'Explanation and social policy: The problem of social inequalities in health', *Journal of Social Policy*, vol. 11, no. 1, pp. 7–32.
Black Report (1980) *Inequalities in Health: Report of a Research Working Group* (London: HMSO).
Blaxter, M. (1981) *The Health of the Children* (London: Heinemann Educational Books).
Blaxter, M. (1983) 'The causes of disease: women talking', *Social Science and Medicine*, vol. 17, no. 2, pp. 54–69.
Blaxter, M. and Paterson, E. (1982) *Mothers and Daughters* (London: Heinemann Educational Books).
Brent Community Health Council (1981) *Black People and the Health Service* (London: Brent Community Health Council).
Brotherston Report (1973) *Towards an Integrated Child Health Service* (Edinburgh: Scottish Home and Health Department).
Burghes, L. (1980) *Living from Hand to Mouth: A Study of 65 Families Living on Supplementary Benefit – Poverty Pamphlet 50* (London: Family Service Units and Child Poverty Action Group).
Burghes, L. (1982) 'Facts and figures', *Poverty* (London: Child Poverty Action Group).
Burnell, I. and Wadsworth, J. (1982) 'Home truths', *One Parent Times*, no. 8, April.

Burnett, J. (1971) *Plenty and Want: A Social History of Diet in England from 1815 to the Present Day* (London: Scolar Press).

Buswell, C. (1983) 'Social acceptability – how mothers perceive normal growth and development in their first child' (Paper given at Medical Sociology Conference, York, September).

Butler, N. R. et al. *From Birth to Five* (Unpublished Report of the Child Health and Education in the Seventies Study. University of Bristol).

Butler, N. R. (1977) 'Family and community influences on 0–5s: utilisation of pre-school day-care and preventive health care' in *Child Health and Education in the Seventies* (Mimeo, The University of Bristol and the National Birthday Trust Fund).

Calnan, M. (1982) 'The hospital accident and emergency department', *Journal of Social Policy*, vol. 11, no. 4, pp. 483–503.

Calnan, M. and Wadsworth, M. (1977) 'Accounting for accidental injury in childhood' in S. Burman and S. Genn (eds) *Accidents in the Home* (London: Croom Helm).

Calnan, M. and Johnson, B. (1985) 'Health, health risks and inequalities: an exploratory study of women's perceptions', *Sociology of Health and Illness*, vol. 7, no. 1.

Cartwright, A. (1967) *Patients and Their Doctors* (London: Routledge & Kegan Paul).

Cartwright, A. and O'Brien, M. (1976) 'Social class variation in health care' in M. Stacey (ed.) *The Sociology of the NHS, Sociological Review Monograph 22* (Keele: University of Keele).

Chalmers, I. (1985) 'Short, Black, Baird, Himsworth, and social class differences in fetal and neonatal mortality rates', *British Medical Journal*, vol. 291, no. 6490, pp. 231–2.

Clark, M. *Training in Health and Race*, 18 Victoria Park Square, London E 2.

Coates, K. and Silburn, R. (1970) *Poverty: The Forgotten Englishmen* (Harmondsworth: Penguin).

Cornwell, J. (1984) *Hard Earned Lives* (London: Tavistock Publications).

Court Report (1976) *Fit For the Future*. The Report of the Committee on Child Health Services, Cmnd 6684 (London: HMSO).

Cowell, C. R. and Sheiham, A. (1981) *Promoting Dental Health* (King Edward's Hospital Fund for London) (London: Pitman Books).

Crawford, R. (1977) 'You are dangerous to your health: the ideology and politics of victim blaming' *International Journal of Health Services*, vol. 7, no. 4, pp. 663–80.

Cunningham-Burley, S. (1984) 'Mothers' perceptions of their children's illnesses: changes in behaviour as problematical concerns' (Paper presented to the BSA Medical Sociology Conference, September).

Davie, R., Butler, N. and Goldstein, H. (1972) *From Birth to Seven: The Second Report of the National Child Development Study* (London: Longmans).

Davis, P. (1980) *The Social Context of Dentistry* (London: Croom Helm).
Department of the Environment (1979) *National Dwelling and Housing Survey* (London: HMSO).
Department of Health and Social Security (1979) *Prevention and Health: Eating for Health* (London: HMSO).
Department of Health and Social Security (1977) *Prevention and Health* (London: HMSO).
Dingwall, R. L. (1982) 'Community nursing and civil liberty', *Journal of Advanced Nursing*, vol. 7, pp. 337–46.
Dingwall, R. and Murray, T. (1983) 'Categorization in accident departments: "good patients", "bad patients" and "children"', *Sociology of Health and Illness*, vol. 5, no. 2, pp. 127–48.
Douglas, J. W. B. and Blomfield, J. M. (1958) *Children Under Five* (London: Allen & Unwin).
Downer, M. C. (1984) 'A review of trends in dental health in the UK', *Journal of the Royal Society of Health*, vol. 104, no. 1, pp. 22–6.
Dunn, J. (1984) *Sisters and Brothers* (London: Fontana Paperbacks).
Dunnell, K. and Dobbs, J. (1982) *Nurses Working in the Community* OPCS (London: HMSO).
Fagin, L. and Little, M. (1984) *The Forsaken Families* (Harmondsworth: Penguin).
Farrant, W. and Russell, J. (1985) *A Case Study in the Production, Distribution and Use of Health Information* Final Report of the Health Education Publications Project (London: Health Education Council).
Farrant, W. and Russell, J. (1986) *Beating Heart Disease: A Case Study in the Production of HEC Publications* (Bedford Way Paper) (London: Institute of Education).
Food Policy Unit (1984) *Jam Tomorrow: A report of the first findings of a pilot study of the food circumstances, attitudes and consumption of 1000 people on low incomes in the North of England* (Manchester: Food Policy Unit).
Freeman, M. (1983) 'Child-rearing: Parental Autonomy and State Intervention' in A. W. Franklin (ed.) *Family Matters* (Oxford: Pergamon Press).
General Medical Services Committee of the BMA (1984) *Handbook of Preventive Care for Pre-School Children* (London: BMA).
Glazer, M. and Moynihan, D. P. (1963) *Beyond the Melting Pot* (Cambridge, Mass.: MIT Press).
Graham, H. (1979) 'Prevention and health: every mother's business. A comment on child health policies in the 1970s' in C. Harris (ed.) *The Sociology of the Family, Sociological Monograph no. 28* (Keele: University of Keele).
Graham, H. (1984) *Women, Health and the Family* (London: Harvester Press).

Graham, H. (1985) *Caring for the Family: A short Report of the Study of the Organisation of Health Resources and Responsibilities in 102 Families with Pre-School children* (Faculty of Social Sciences, Open University, unpublished report).

Graham, H. and McKee, L. (1980) *The First Months of Motherhood: Report of a Survey of Women's Experiences of Pregnancy, Childbirth and the First Six Months after Birth* (London: Health Education Council).

Greater London Council (1980) *A Social Review of Greater London, Reviews and Studies no. 3* (London: Greater London Council).

Hall, P. and Lawrence, S. (1981) 'Deprivation in the Inner City' in P. Hall (ed.) *The Inner City in Context: The Final Report of the Social Science Research Council Inner Cities Working Party* (London: Heinemann Educational Books).

Harris, C. (ed.) *The Sociology of the Family, Sociological Monograph no. 28* (Keele: University of Keele).

Harrison, P. (1983) *Inside the Inner City* (Harmondsworth: Penguin).

Health Education Council (1978) *The Scientific Basis of Dental Health Education: A Policy Statement* (London: Health Education Council).

Health Education Council (undated) *Is This What you Want for Your Child?* HEC.

Health Education Council (undated) *Diet and Healthy Teeth* HEC.

Health Education Council (undated) *The Six-Year Molars* HEC.

Health Education Council (undated) *Immunisation* Health Education Council leaflet.

Health Education Council (undated) *Measles is Misery* Health Education Council leaflet.

Health Visitors Association (1981) *Health Visiting in the 80s* Health Visitors Association.

Helman, C. G. (1984) *Culture Health and Illness: An Introduction for Health Professionals* (Bristol: Wright).

Hendrickse, W. A. (1982) 'How effective are our child health clinics?' *British Medical Journal*, vol. 284, pp. 575–7.

Herzlich, C. (1973) *Health and Illness: A Social Psychological Analysis* (London: Academic Press).

Hoggart, R. (1958) *The Uses of Literacy* (Harmondsworth: Penguin).

Hughes, M., Mayall, B., Moss, P., Perry, J., Petrie, P. and Pinkerton, G. (1980) *Nurseries Now* (Harmondsworth: Penguin).

Hull, D. (1981) 'Interpretation of the contraindications to whooping cough vaccination' *British Medical Journal*, vol. 283, pp. 1231–3.

Ineichen, B. (1979) 'Housing factors in the timing of weddings and first pregnancies' in *The Sociology of the Family: New Directions for Britain, Sociological Review Monograph, no. 28* (Keele: University of Keele).

Jefferys, M. and Sachs, H. (1983) *Rethinking General Practice* (London: Tavistock Publications).

Joffe, M. and Grisso, J. E. (1985) 'Comparison of ante-natal hospital records with retrospective interviewing', *Journal of Biosocial Science*, vol. 17, pp. 113–119.

Jolly, H. (1981) *Book of Child Care: The Complete Guide for Today's Parents* (London: Sphere Books).

Jones, A. E. (1984) 'Domiciliary immunisation for preschool child defaulters' *British Medical Journal*, vol. 289, pp. 1429–31.

Jones, K., Brown, J. and Bradshaw, J. (1983) 'Two nations?' in *Issues in Social Policy* (London: Routledge & Kegan Paul).

Jones, K., Brown, J., Bradshaw, J. (1983) *Issues in Social Policy* (2nd edn.) (Routledge & Kegan Paul).

Kamerman, S. B. and Kahn, A. J. (eds) *Child Care, Family Benefits and Working Parents: A Study in Family Policy* (New York: Columbia University Press).

Kerr, M. and Charles, N. (1984) *Attitudes Towards the Feeding and Nutrition of Young Children: First Report of a Health Education Council Project into Family Feeding Practices* (unpublished).

King, J. (1984) 'A multi-disciplinary approach', *Nursing Times*, vol. 80, no. 27, pp. 32–3.

Kruk, S. and Wolkind, S. (1983) 'A Longitudinal Study of Single Mothers and their children' in N. Madge (ed.) *Families at Risk* (London: Heinemann Educational Books).

Lawrence, D. (1980) 'Race, immigration and the new rules' in *Patterns of Prejudice* (London: Institute of Jewish Affairs).

Leach, E. (1983) 'Are there alternatives to the family' in A. W. Franklin (ed.) *Family Matters* (Harmondsworth: Penguin).

Leach, P. (1977) *Baby and Child: From Birth to Age Five* (Harmondsworth: Penguin).

Leete, R. and Fox, J. (1977) Registrar General Social Classes: Origins and Uses, *Population Trends 8*, OPCS. (London: HMSO).

Lewis, J. (1980) *The Politics of Motherhood* (London: Croom Helm).

Lewis, O. (1963) *The Children of Sanchez* (London: Vintage Books).

Lobstein, T. and Sheiham, A. (1980) *The User's View of Dental Services* (London: Department of Community Dental Health, London Hospital Medical College).

Locker, D. (1980) *Symptoms and Illness* (London: Tavistock Publications).

Luker, K. (1975) *Taking Chances: Abortion and the Decision not to Contracept* (Berkeley, CA: University of California Press).

Madge, N. (1983) 'Unemployment and its effects on children', *Journal of Child Psychology and Psychiatry*, vol. 24, no. 2, pp. 311–19.

Mayall, M. and Grossmith, C. (1984) *Caring for the Health of Young Children* Report to the ESRC, August 1984 (London: Economic and Social Research Council).

Mayall, B. and Petrie, P. (1983) *Childminding and Day Nurseries: What*

Kind of Care? Studies in Education, 13. (London: Heinemann Educational Books, for the Institute of Education).

Macfarlane, J. A. and Pillay, U. (1984) 'Who does what and how much in the preschool child health services in England', *British Medical Journal*, vol. 289, pp. 851–2.

Medical Market Information Ltd (1982) *The Directory of Health Centres* (London: MMI).

McNay, M. and Pond, C. (1980) *Low pay and family poverty* (London: Study Commission on the Family, 231 Baker Street, London NW1 6XL).

McGuire, J. (1983) *The Effect of a Child's Gender on the Nature of Parent-Child Interactions in the Home, During the Third Year of Life* (London: University of London PhD thesis).

Moss, P. (1976) 'Current issues' in N. Fonda and P. Moss (eds) 'Mothers in Employment', Papers from a Conference on Mothers in Employment: Trends and Issues (Uxbridge: Brunel University).

Moss, P. (1985) 'Some principles for a childcare service for working parents', Paper presented at EOC Workshop on Childcare Policy (London: Institute of Education).

Moss, P., Bolland, G., and Foxman, R. (1982) *Transition to Parenthood* Report to DHSS.

Murcott, A. (1983) (ed.) *The Sociology of Food and Eating* (Aldershot: Gower Press).

National Advisory Committee on Nutrition Education (NACNE) (1983) *A discussion paper on proposals for nutritional guidelines for health education in Britain* (London: Health Education Council).

Newson, J. and Newson, E. (1970) *Four Years Old in an Urban Community* (Harmondsworth: Penguin).

Newson, J. and Newson, E. (1965) *Patterns of Infant Care in an Urban Community* (Harmondsworth: Penguin).

Newson, J. and Newson, E. (1978) *Seven Years Old in the Home Environment* (Harmondsworth: Penguin Books).

Nicoll, A. (1983) 'Community child health services – for better or worse', *Health Visitor*, vol. 56, no. 7, pp. 241–3.

Nicoll, A. (1985) 'Contraindications to whooping cough immunisation – myths or realities?', *The Lancet*, vol. i, pp. 679–81.

Office of Health Economics (1981) *Accidents in Childhood* (Briefing no. 17) (London: OHE).

Office of Health Economics (1984) *Childhood Vaccination: Current Controversies* (London: OHE).

OPCS (1983) *General Household Survey, 1981* (London: HMSO).

OPCS (1984a) *General Household Survey, (1982)* (London: HMSO).

OPCS (1984b) *Infant and Perinatal Mortality, 1982* OPCS Monitor DH3 84/6 (London: HMSO).

OPCS (1985) *Infant and Perinatal Mortality* (1983): birthweight. OPCS Monitor DH3 85/1 (London: HMSO).

Orr, J. (1980) *Health Visiting in focus: a Consumer's View of Health Visiting in Northern Ireland* (London: Royal College of Nursing).

Osborn, A. F. and Morris, T. C. (1979) 'The rationale for a composite index of social class and its evaluation', *British Journal of Sociology*, vol. 30, no. 1, pp. 39–60.

Osborn, A. F. and Butler, N. R. (1985) *Ethnic Minority Children: A Comparative Study From Birth to Five Years* (London: Commission for Racial Equality).

Pattison, C. J., Drinkwater, C. K. and Downham, M. P. S. (1982) 'Mothers' appreciation of their children's symptoms', *Journal of the Royal College of General Practitioners*, March, pp. 149–62.

Piachaud, D. (1981a) *Round About Fifty Hours A Week: the time costs of children* (London: Child Poverty Action Group).

Piachaud, D. (1981b) *Children and Poverty* (Poverty Research Series, no. 9, Dec.) (London: Child Poverty Action Group).

Philp, A. F. (1963) *Family Failure: a Study of 129 Families with Multiple Problems* (London: Faber & Faber).

Pill, R. and Stott, N. (1983) 'Concepts of illness causation and responsibility: some preliminary data from a sample of working class mothers', *Social Science and Medicine*, vol. 16, no. 1, pp. 43–52.

Polgar, S. (1963) 'Health action in cross-cultural perspectives' in H. E. Freeman, S. Levine and L. G. Reeder (eds) *Handbook of Medical Sociology* (Englewood Cliffs, N.J.: Prentice-Hall).

Polnay, L. (1985) 'The community paediatric team – an approach to child health services in a deprived inner city area' in J. A. MacFarlane (ed.) *Progress in Child Health*, vol. I (Edinburgh: Churchill Livingstone).

Ross, E. M., Peckham, C. S., West, P. B. and Butler, N. R. (1980) 'Epilepsy in childhood: findings from the National Child Development Study', *British Medical Journal*, vol. 280, pp. 207–10.

Royal College of General Practitioners (1981) *Health and Prevention in Primary Care* (London: RCGP).

Royal College of General Practitioners (1982) *Healthier Children – Thinking Prevention* (London: RCGP).

Royal College of General Practitioners (1984) *Handbook of Preventive Care for Pre-School Children* (London: RCGP).

Russan, A. (1977) 'The Psychology of Children in Traffic' in R. H. Jackson (ed.) *Children, the Environment and Accidents* (London: Pitmans Medical Publications).

Sinnott, W. R. (1977) 'Safety aspects of domestic architecture' in R. H. Jackson (ed.) *Children, the Environment and Accidents* (London: Pitmans Medical Publications).

Skrimshire, A. (1978) *Area Disadvantage, Social Class and The Health*

Service (Oxford: Social Evaluation Unit, Department of Social and Administrative Studies).

Smith, A. (1970) *The Body* (Harmondsworth: Penguin Books).

Spence, J., Walton, W. S., Miller, F. J. W. and Court, S. D. M. (1954) *A Thousand Families in Newcastle upon Tyne: an Approach to the Study of Health and Illness in Children* (London: Oxford University Press).

Spencer, N. J. (1984) 'Patients' recognition of the ill child' in J. A. MacFarlane (ed.) *Progress in Child Health*, vol. 1 (London: Churchill Livingstone).

Spring-Rice, M. (1939) *Working Class Wives* (Harmondsworth: Penguin. Republished 1981, London: Virago).

Stacey, M. and Davies, C. (1983) *Division of Labour in Child Health Care: final Report to the SSRC* (Warwick: University of Warwick).

Steiner, H. (1977) 'An evaluation of child health clinic services in Newcastle upon Tyne during 1972–1974', *British Journal of Preventive and Social Medicine*, vol. 31, no. 1, pp. 1–5.

Strong, P. M. (1979) 'Sociological imperialism and the profession of medicine', *Social Science and Medicine*. vol. 13A, no. 2, pp. 199–215.

Thomson, J. D. (1984) *In Camden Town* (Harmondsworth: Penguin).

Todd, J. E. and Todd, T. (1985) *Children's Dental Health in the United Kingdom 1983*: A survey carried out by the Social Survey Division of OPCS, on behalf of the UK Health Departments, in collaboration with the Dental Schools of the Universities of Birmingham and Newcastle. OPCS Series SS 1189 (London: HMSO).

Townsend, P. and Davidson, N. (1982) *Inequalities in Health: The Black Report* (Harmondsworth: Penguin).

Townsend, P., Simpson, D. and Tibbs, N. (1984) *Inequalities of Health in the City of Bristol* (Bristol: Department of Social Administration, University of Bristol).

Tonge, W. L., James, D. S. and Hillam, S. M. (1975) *Families Without Hope* (Ashford, Kent: Headley Bros. Ltd).

Tudor Hart, J. (1971) 'The inverse care law', *Lancet*, vol. 1, p. 405.

Webber, R. (1977) *National Classification of Residential Neighbourhoods* (London: Planning Research Applications Group).

Wilding, P. (1982) *Professional Power and Social Welfare* (London: Routledge & Kegan Paul).

Williams, A. S. and Fairpo, C. G. (1984) 'Health visitors and dental health awareness', *Midwife, Health Visitor and Community Nurse*, vol. 20, no. 2, pp. 45–50.

Williams, P. R. (1983) 'Does your child health clinic meet the needs of mothers as well as children?', *Journal of the Royal College of General Practitioners*, vol. 33, p. 505.

Wilson, H. and Herbert, G. W. (1978) *Parents and Children in the Inner City* (London: Routledge & Kegan Paul).